MUSCLE BIOPSY

Edited by **Challa Sundaram**

Muscle Biopsy
Edited by Challa Sundaram

Published by InTech

Janeza Trdine 9, 51000 Rijeka, Croatia

Publishing Process Manager Oliver Kurelic

Technical Editor Teodora Smiljanic

Cover Designer InTech Design Team

Additional hard copies can be obtained from orders@intechopen.com

Muscle Biopsy, Edited Challa Sundaram
p. cm.
ISBN 978-953-307-778-9

For EU product safety concerns:
IN TECH d.o.o., Prolaz Marije Krucifikse Kozulić 3, 51000 Rijeka, Croatia,
info@intechopen.com or visit our website at intechopen.com.

Meet the editor

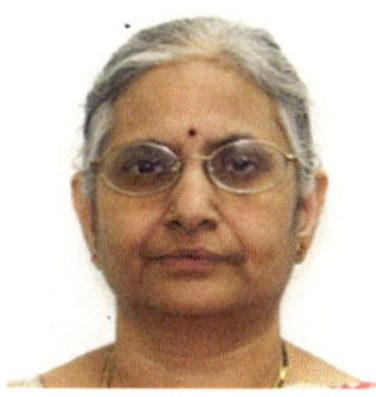

Senior Professor and Head, Department of Pathology, Nizam's Institute of Medical Sciences, Hyderabad, Andhra Pradesh, India. She did her MD Pathology at Andhra University, Visakhapatnam, Andhra Pradesh. She had her training in Neuropathology at Southern General Hospital, Glasgow, UK. She established the neuropathology services in her laboratory in the state of Andhra Pradesh and is actively involved in the diagnosis of Neurooncology, Neuroinfections and neuromuscular diseases. She published a large series of mitochondrial myopathies with particular emphasis on chronic progressive external opthalmoplegia on muscle biopsy and genetics. Her other contributions include proteomic studies in human gliomas and CNS fungal infections.

Contents

Preface

With this book, 'Muscle Biopsy', I published my first book as an editor on diagnostic issues of muscle biopsies - the work which I have cherished for the last 25 years. The use and importance of doing and interpreting a muscle biopsy has come a long way after the first biopsy was performed by Duchenne to diagnose a myopathic condition. Starting as a relatively less attractive field, myology, particularly myopathology, has progressed into one of the most coveted subjects by neurologists, pathologists and basic scientists. With advances in enzyme histochemistry, molecular pathology and gene analysis, the importance of a muscle biopsy in the diagnosis of primary and secondary neuromuscular disorders is increasing.

The diagnostic algorithm on a muscle biopsy begins with a systematic and thorough analysis of histochemical and enzyme histochemical stains. The first two chapters of the book deal with these basics of muscle biopsy. The next set of two chapters deals with basic research techniques of cultures of myotubes and membrane transport. These chapters give an in-depth review of basic techniques seldom covered in any other book on muscle biopsy and will be of great help to basic scientists.

Mitochondrial disease pathology and pathogenesis has made tremendous progress over the last few years and has given answers to many unexplained neuromuscular and systemic ailments. Mitochondria have also established a role in pathogenesis of diabetes and obesity. Keeping this in mind, we have included three chapters which deal with different aspects of mitochondrial diseases.

I am greatly thankful to all the authors of this book for their contributions and hope the readers benefit from the material.

Challa Sundaram
Department of Pathology,
Nizam's Institute of Medical Sciences, Hyderabad,
India

Part 1

Muscle Biopsy: Procedure and Interpretation

1

Percutaneous Muscle Biopsy: History, Methods and Acceptability

Harnish P. Patel, Cyrus Cooper and Avan Aihie Sayer
MRC Lifecourse Epidemiology Unit, University of Southampton, Southampton UK

1. Introduction

Advances in histological, biochemical, physiological and molecular biological assays, as well as in microscopy and image analysis have allowed multiple analyses in muscle tissue (1-5). Muscle biopsy is invaluable in providing a definitive diagnosis of a wide range of myopathies (muscular dystrophies, glycogen storage diseases, inflammatory myopathies and congenital myopathies) and denervating disorders and gives important information on the course of the disease, informs treatment, disease stage as well as prognosis. Results of histopathological analyses should then be interpreted in context of the clinical history, examination and laboratory serum markers (1;6). Furthermore, access to muscle tissue provides the opportunity to assess morphological characteristics such as fibre composition, fibre cross sectional area and capillarisation (e.g. in ageing muscle) (7-9) as well as mRNA, protein abundance and muscle enzyme activity (10). Ultrastructural analyses to gauge response to intervention can be performed (11) as can studies of physiological characteristics of muscle such as single fibre contraction properties (2;8).

2. History of muscle biopsy

Methodologies enabling the study of muscle tissue have relied on obtaining tissue through post mortem or open muscle biopsy techniques that require general anaesthesia. Although open muscle biopsy provides large specimens that enables direct visualization of disease distribution and can include a peripheral nerve, the technique involves co-ordination between surgical and anaesthetic colleagues, requires an inpatient bed stay and is therefore time and resource demanding. Moreover, this technique can result in significant scarring.

Microscopic analysis of muscle obtained through percutaneous biopsy can be credited to the French Neurologist Guillaume-Benjamin-Amand Duchenne (1806-1875), lauded for describing muscular dystrophy amongst his many other accolades. Fuelled by his passionate interest in muscular diseases and electrophysiology, he constructed a needle possessing a trocar that made it possible to obtain muscle tissue and was the first clinician to perform percutaneous or 'semi-open' muscle biopsy in living subjects without anaesthesia (12).

Numerous muscle biopsy needles have since been described (13;14). However, the percutaneous needle introduced by Bergstrom in 1962 (15), similar in characteristic to the needle described by Duchenne, gained popularity through widespread use in diagnostic as well as research (study of normal muscle in relation to physiological change) purposes in both children and adults (3;4;16). Although continuously being refined (17;18), each iteration of the needle is true to its origins i.e. possess a sharp trocar, a cutting cannula that needs sharpening perhaps every 10 uses and a pushing rod to expel the tissue post biopsy (Figure 1). Muscle yields obtained from the needle biopsy have been reported to vary from 25-75 mg (2) 70 - 140mg (4) and up to 143-293 mg after repeated sampling (19).

An alternative instrument to the Bergstrom biopsy needle is the Weil-Blakesley conchotome (Figure 2) (20-22). This instrument, designed like a forcep was described by Henriksson in 1979 (21) and consists of a sharp biting tip encompassing a hollow that can vary from 4-6 mm in width. In similar fashion to the Bergstrom needle, it is inserted through a skin incision 5-10mm in length but does not require a sharp trocar to aid muscle penetration. In addition, its design allows controlled tissue penetration and offers a degree of manoeuvrability (22). These features allow biopsy on a wider range of muscles and permits sampling of muscle groups where the pressure required for the needle procedure to penetrate muscle may not be advisable because of overlying neurovascular or underlying bony structures e.g. at the tibialis anterior (22;23). An additional benefit is that, unlike the Bergstrom needle, the conchotome biting tip does not need regular sharpening and has been reported to maintain sharpness for up to 4 years (17). Muscle yields from the conchotome technique in the earliest report by Henriksson (21) ranged from 26 to 296mg. In our practice, muscle weights ranged at a comparable 20-290mg (24).

3. Micro-biopsy

The 'semi-open' techniques described above requiring an incision may be considered too painful and the potential for scarring may be off putting for some. Furthermore, semi-open techniques may be impractical to study time course responses to intervention e.g. exercise or drug administration. As a consequence, minimally invasive techniques such as micro-biopsy have been explored (19;25;26). The device used for skeletal muscle micro-biopsy is a version of the popular spring loaded one-handed automated biopsy systems used to perform biopsies of the breast, prostate, kidney or liver. The assembly consists of a disposable core biopsy needle e.g. 16G Magnum ® (Bard Ltd, UK) and an insertion cannula that will allow multiple biopsies to be performed via a single insertion site (Figure 3). The needle penetration depth can be pre-set by the operator after which release of a trigger unloads the spring and fires the needle into the muscle, excising a small piece of tissue. The validity of this method compared with the Bergstrom needle in histomorphometric analyses has been tested (19).

The semi-open muscle biopsy and micro-biopsy techniques are common, simple and easily learned procedures that have superseded open muscle biopsy in clinical as well as research practice (4;6;17). Any potential risks are reduced if performed correctly and with strict attention to asepsis. Muscles that can be subject to biopsy include the deltoid, biceps, triceps, tibialis anterior, gastrocnemius, soleus and the sacrospinal muscles (3;22;23;27;28). However, the most common site for biopsy both in clinical and research practice is the outermost portion of the *vastus lateralis*. This site, approximately two-thirds down a line from the anterior superior iliac spine to the patella is readily accessible and does not contain an overlying neurovascular bundle. Furthermore, extensive normative fibre histo-morphometric data obtained from vastus lateralis biopsy exists in the literature that allows the recognition of normal and abnormal and facilitates comparison between studies (2;6).

4. Vastus lateralis muscle biopsy (Figure 4)

The biopsy technique using the Weil-Blakesley conchotome and the Bergstrom needle is described below. The technique for micro-biopsy is reviewed by Hayot et al (19); apart from the fact that a skin incision is not required, the procedure shares the same principle as for the conchotome and needle methods and is illustrated in Figure 5.

Equipment needed for percutaneous muscle biopsy

1. Weil-Blakesley conchotome with either 4mm or 6mm biting tip (*Gebrüder Zepf Medizintechnik, Dürbheim, Germany*) (Figure 2) or Bergstrom needle with either 4mm or 6mm cutting trocar (*Dixons surgical instruments Ltd, UK*) (Figure 1)
2. 10ml and 20ml syringes
3. Scalpel size 11
4. Sterile gauze squares and sterile saline-soaked gauze squares
5. Sterile drape with adhesive aperture (*Steri-Drape* ™, *3M Health Care, USA*)
6. Chlorhexidine or iodine based skin disinfectant
7. 5-10ml 2% Lidocaine without epinephrine
8. Sterile 10ml Universal Container
9. Quarter inch steri-strips
10. Stretchable bandage and elastic tape for compression
11. Ice

Optional (dependent on planned analyses)

1. Liquid nitrogen and suitable cryovials
2. Isopentane cooled in liquid nitrogen
3. Cork disc
4. OTC mount
5. Fixative e.g. formalin, 3% Glutaralhedyde/4% formaldehyde
6. Dissecting microscope to orientate tissue sample so that sections with fibres in true cross-section can be obtained
7. Suitable blunt edged forceps for post procedure tissue handling

In the clinical setting, muscle biopsies are conducted based on patient symptoms and the distribution of muscular weakness and generally do not require standardised conditions but do require the biopsy site to be free of previous muscle injury, contractures or prior instrumentation/therapy e.g. injection sites (1;6). In research or in quantitative studies, standard conditions should apply to all procedures. For example, studies may require participants to be fasted pre biopsy or the exclusion of diabetic subjects (24).

There is little guidance on the use of aspirin or other anti-platelet agents pre biopsy. Whereas warfarin and related anticoagulants would need to be stopped for at least one to two weeks prior to the procedure, aspirin was stopped 4-7 days prior to uneventful muscle

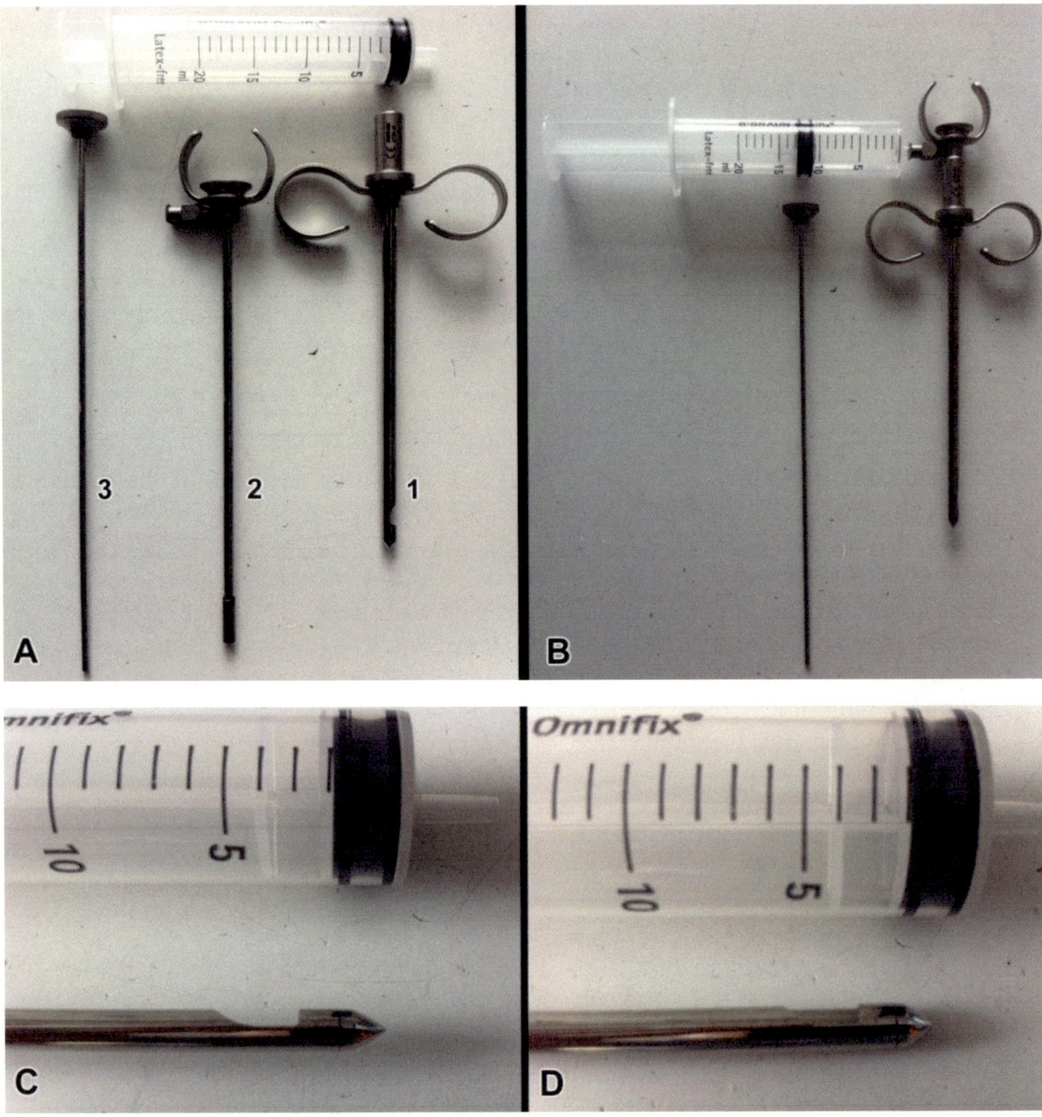

Fig. 1. A. Components of the biopsy needle include 1. Trocar, 2. Cutting cannula, 3. Clearing probe/rod. B. Assembled for biopsy, with cutting cannula inserted within the trocar. A 20 ml syringe can be connected to the cutting cannula to increase the yield of tissue by suction. C. Cutting window visible. D. Window with cutting cannula fully depressed.

biopsy in our research study (24). It is likely that the drug free duration would need to be longer for ADP receptor blockers e.g. clopidogrel. Obviously, risks of stopping such secondary prevention drugs must be considered case-by-case.

Participants are asked to lay supine, comfortably on a bed with the preferred thigh exposed from the groin crease. The operator should be positioned adjacent to the thigh however, a position adjacent to the contra-lateral thigh with the operator reaching over can also be assumed according to individual preference. The leg should remain straight and relaxed

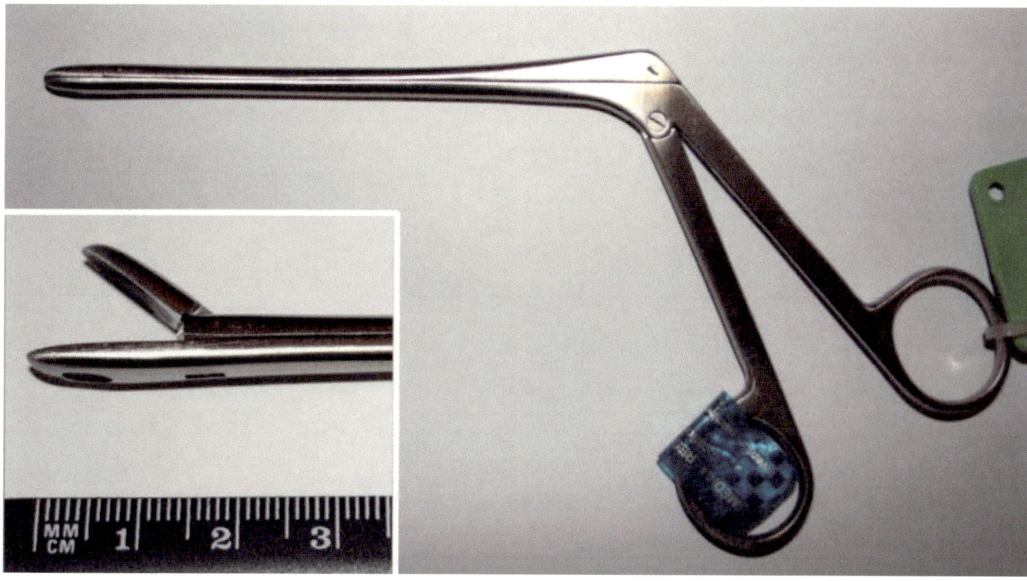

Fig. 2. The Weil-Blakelsley Cochotome with a 6mm bitting tip (*From Patel HP et al [24]*)

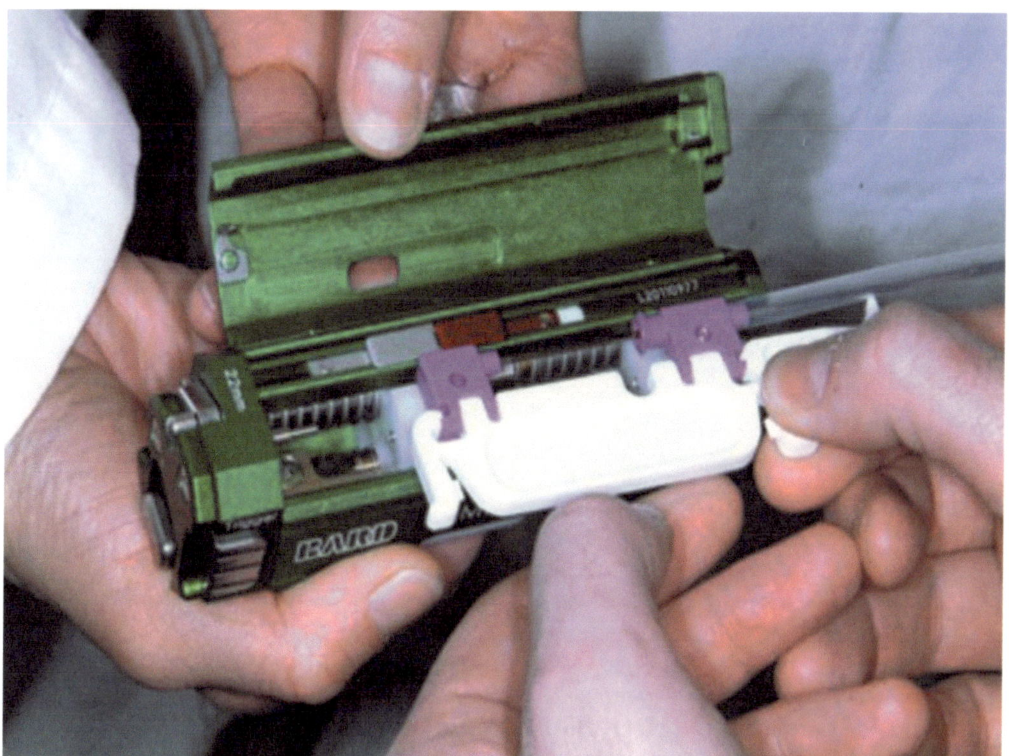

Fig. 3. Spring loaded micro-biopsy system consisting of trigger housing, biopsy needle and the insertion cannula (not shown). (*Illustration kindly provided by M Hayot, Service Central de Physiologie Clinique, Montpellier, France*)

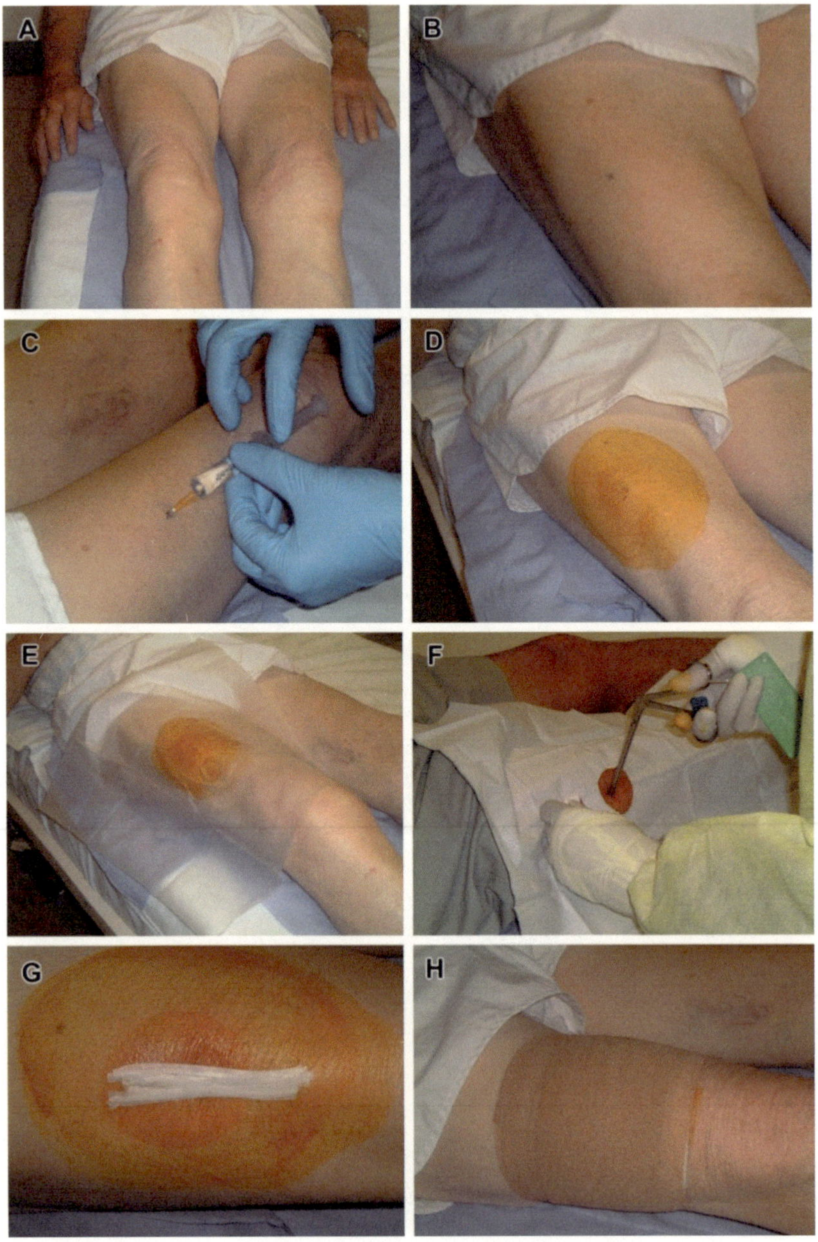

A. The leg is exposed from the groin crease down to the ankle. B The biopsy area, approximately 2/3 down a line from the anterior superior iliac spine to the patella is marked. C&D The biopsy site over the vastus lateralis is shaved of hair, infiltrated with local anaesthetic and cleaned with antiseptic. E. The biopsy site is isolated with a sterile drape that has a 10 cm adhesive aperture. F. The skin and overlying fascia is then punctured with a size 11 scalpel. The conchotome tip is inserted into the track made by the scalpel, opened, closed and rotated through 90° to excise tissue. G&H. The 5-10mm wound is closed with steri-strips after which a dry dressing and compression bandage are applied.

Fig. 4. The muscle biopsy procedure using the Weil-Blakesley conchotome

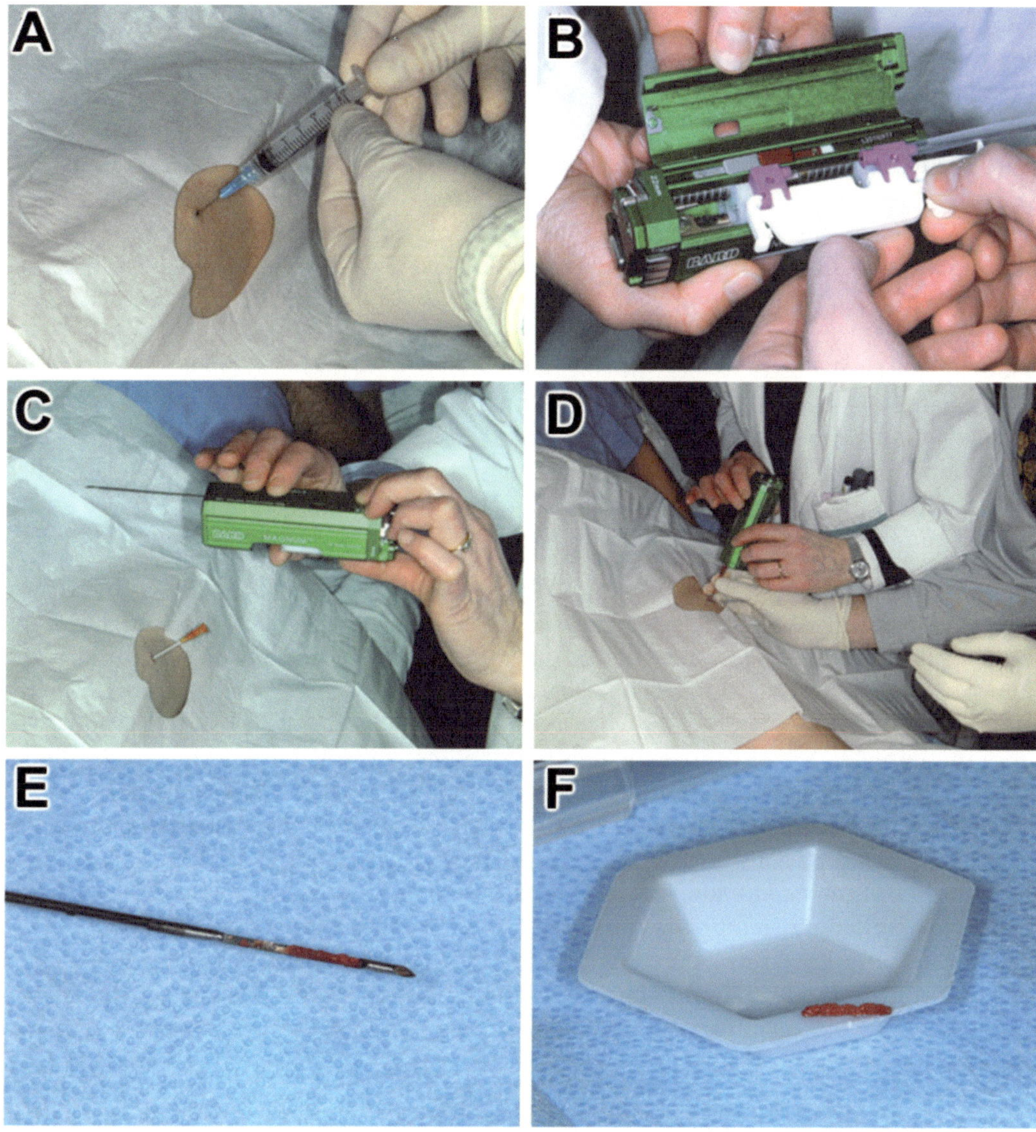

A. Infiltration with local anaesthesia. B. Placement of biopsy needle into the trigger housing. C. Skin puncture with the insertion cannula. D. Insertion of the biopsy needle through the insertion cannula and trigger release. E. Removal of the of the muscle specimen aided by a sterile scalpel (insertion cannula can remain in situ to permit repeated sampling). F. Weighing of the sample. (Reproduced with permission of the European Respiratory Society ©)

Fig. 5. Micro-biopsy procedure with the Magnum ® biopsy system (Bard Ltd, UK)[19]

throughout the procedure but the thigh can be tensed momentarily to accentuate the outline of the vastus lateralis to mark the biopsy site. Thereafter the skin surrounding the mark is shaved and cleaned with an alcohol swab.

The skin and overlying fascia is then infiltrated with 5mls of 2% lidocaine local anaesthetic. The subcutaneous bleb is allowed to dissipate during which time the operator should dawn a sterile gown, gloves and create a sterile field on a suitable trolley. After opening the pack containing the Conchotome or biopsy needle, the skin should be sterilized with povidone iodine *(Betadine) or a 2%* Chlorhexidine gluconate/isopropyl alcohol solution according to local infection control protocols. A sterile drape with an adhesive aperture is then used to maintain a sterile field. With a size 11 scalpel, a 5-10mm incision is made on the skin and down to the fascia through which the closed biting tip of the conchotome is inserted. The conchotome is inserted at right angles to the long axis of the femur, facing away from the femur and to a depth averaging 2-5cm. The free hand of the operator can hold the thigh surrounding the biopsy site while the tip of the conchotome is opened and closed (scissor action) to interpose muscle tissue. The conchotome is then rotated through 90-180° to cut the muscle. Sampling takes a few seconds and can be repeated within the single site, where necessary, to obtain sufficient muscle tissue given the high probability of sampling adipose tissue initially (Figure 4 A-H). The biopsies should be placed on sterile saline-dampened gauze and then transferred into a universal container or petri dish and placed on ice for the remainder of the procedure.

Operator and skin preparation prior to using the using the needle biopsy or the micro-biopsy gun is exactly the same as described for the conchotome (17;29). Constituents of the needle include include the trocar/needle, the cutting cannula and the clearing probe/rod (Figure 1A 1,2,3 respectively). The instrument should be assembled by inserting the cutting cannula into the trocar and checked to ensure alignment and sliding action. The width of a size 11 scalpel to make a skin incision and a track down to the fascia should suffice. The trocar is inserted through the incision, past the fascia where the operator should get a sensation of overcoming resistance; at this point the window of the trocar (Figure 1C) should be fully in the muscle. The cutting cannula is withdrawn a few centimetres and the needle angled to allow tissue to enter the instrument. Alternatively, an assistant can apply suction via a syringe applied to the cutting cannula (Figure 1B) to draw muscle into the cutting chamber before fully advancing the cannula to guillotine a section of muscle (18;30) (Figure 1D) The free hand of the operator can be used to steady the thigh. The yield of muscle can be increased by rotating the instrument by 90° and repeating the procedure (18).

Post procedure, direct pressure should be applied to the wound for 5-10 minutes prior to closure with steri-strips (*Leukostrip, Smith and Nephew, UK*). Sterile absorbent gauze is placed on the steri-strips and a clear adhesive film (*Bioclusive™, Johnson and Johnson, UK*) placed on the gauze. A two-layer compression bandage is then tied for up to 6 hours. The subject is asked to lay down for up to half an hour post procedure and is observed. The procedure, using the conchotome or the Bergstrom needle can take between 15 and 20 minutes; the majority of said time spent in preparation.

4.1 Post muscle biopsy patient/participant advice

Following the procedure it is common to experience some thigh stiffness that can be alleviated by gentle exercise e.g. walking. There are no real restrictions to mobility but in our practice we ask participants to avoid 1. vigorous activity for 72 hours (hill climbing, running, heavy lifting) and 2. Immersion in water for 48-72 hours (24). Participants can shower if the biopsy site was protected from water for example, wrapping polythene plastic/cling film around the thigh. Written instructions for post biopsy care, spare dressings and emergency contact details should be given to each participant or patient. To ensure full wound healing, that can take up to two weeks, the dressing should be changed after 4 days and steri-strips removed at day 7 post procedure. All those having the procedure should be warned about transient numbness around the biopsy site that may persist for up to two weeks as well as the remote possibility of wound infection that would necessitate a medical consult.

5. Acceptability and adverse events

When performed correctly and according to protocol, the semi-open and micro-biopsy techniques result only in minor discomfort for the subject that is qualitatively described as a "pushing sensation" or a "deep pressure" (29) with very low pain scores (Table 1) (24). Post biopsy, there may be local soreness, stiffness or cramp that do not seem to limit normal activity including recreational sports e.g. golf, bowls (18;24) (Table 1). One participant in our research study reported running a Marathon two weeks after a conchotome vastus lateralis biopsy (24).

Where authors have reported complications, they have commonly been wound haematomas (4;20;22;26). For example, a subject had been taking aspirin at the time of the

VAS pain score (mm)	Median (IQR)
During the procedure	7(1-34)
1 day post procedure	4(0-16)
7 days post procedure	1(0-4)
Daily activity resumed	N (%)
After one day	60(65%)
After 2 days	26(28%)
>2 days	7 (7%)

Table 1. Pain visual analogue scale (VAS) score and resumption of daily activity in 93 research participants subject to the conchotome muscle biopsy. Pain scale was marked at 0mm -'no pain' and at 100mm – 'pain as bad as it can be'. Typically pain scores were low during and post procedure. The majority of the participants resumed daily activity one-day post procedure (*Adapted from Patel HP et al [24]*)

biopsy (20) or did not follow post biopsy recommendations and put an undue amount of strain onto the thigh shortly after the procedure (22). Pain only occurs if the fascia is caught in the needle or a nerve is sampled inadvertently and may persist for one to two weeks (6). There have been no reports in the literature of serious wound infections or disability post procedure.

Minimally invasive muscle biopsy techniques described above are both feasible and acceptable in clinical and research practice with good safety profiles. The choice of instrument depends on experience and preference, tissue requirement, location of muscle as well as clinical assessment of disease involvement. When performed correctly, all yield muscle tissue satisfactory for most histochemical and histological analyses. In addition, the semi-open techniques allow detailed morphological, biochemical and molecular biological analyses to be conducted on muscle tissue.

6. References

[1] Anderson JR. Recommendations for the biopsy procedure and assessment of skeletal muscle biopsies. Virchows Arch 1997 Oct;431(4):227-33.

[2] Coggan AR. Muscle biopsy as a tool in the study of aging. J Gerontol A Biol Sci Med Sci 1995 Nov;50 Spec No:30-4.

[3] Edwards R, Young A, Wiles M. Needle biopsy of skeletal muscle in the diagnosis of myopathy and the clinical study of muscle function and repair. N Engl J Med 1980 Jan 31;302(5):261-71.

[4] Edwards RH, Round JM, Jones DA. Needle biopsy of skeletal muscle: a review of 10 years experience. Muscle Nerve 1983 Nov;6(9):676-83.

[5] Giresi PG, Stevenson EJ, Theilhaber J, Koncarevic A, Parkington J, Fielding RA, et al. Identification of a molecular signature of sarcopenia. Physiol Genomics 2005 Apr 14;21(2):253-63.

[6] Dubowitz V, Sewry C A. Muscle Biopsy: A Practical Approach. 3rd ed ed. China: Saunders Elsevier; 2007.

[7] Charifi N, Kadi F, Feasson L, Costes F, Geyssant A, Denis C. Enhancement of microvessel tortuosity in the vastus lateralis muscle of old men in response to endurance training. J Physiol 2004 Jan 15;554(Pt 2):559-69.

[8] Frontera WR, Suh D, Krivickas LS, Hughes VA, Goldstein R, Roubenoff R. Skeletal muscle fiber quality in older men and women. Am J Physiol Cell Physiol 2000 Sep;279(3):C611-C618.

[9] Patel H, Jameson K, Syddall H, Martin H, Stewart C, Cooper C, et al. Developmental Influences, Muscle Morphology, and Sarcopenia in Community-Dwelling Older Men. J Gerontol A Biol Sci Med Sci 2011 Feb 28.

[10] Costill DL, Daniels J, Evans W, Fink W, Krahenbuhl G, Saltin B. Skeletal muscle enzymes and fiber composition in male and female track athletes. J Appl Physiol 1976 Feb;40(2):149-54.

[11] Sinha-Hikim I, Cornford M, Gaytan H, Lee ML, Bhasin S. Effects of testosterone supplementation on skeletal muscle fiber hypertrophy and satellite cells in community-dwelling older men. J Clin Endocrinol Metab 2006 Aug;91(8):3024-33.

[12] Charriere M, Duchenne GB. Emporte piece histologique. Bull Acad Med 1865;30:1050-1.
[13] O'Rourke KS, Blaivas M, Ike RW. Utility of needle muscle biopsy in a university rheumatology practice. J Rheumatol 1994 Mar;21(3):413-24.
[14] O'Rourke KS, Ike RW. Muscle biopsy. Curr Opin Rheumatol 1995 Nov;7(6):462-8.
[15] Bergstrom J. Muscle electrolytes in man. Scand J Clin Lab Invest 1962;14(suppl. 68).
[16] Edwards RH. Percutaneous needle-biopsy of skeletal muscle in diagnosis and research. Lancet 1971 Sep 11;2(7724):593-5.
[17] Dietrichson P, Coakley J, Smith PE, Griffiths RD, Helliwell TR, Edwards RH. Conchotome and needle percutaneous biopsy of skeletal muscle. J Neurol Neurosurg Psychiatry 1987 Nov;50(11):1461-7.
[18] Hennessey JV, Chromiak JA, Della VS, Guertin J, MacLean DB. Increase in percutaneous muscle biopsy yield with a suction-enhancement technique. J Appl Physiol 1997 Jun;82(6):1739-42.
[19] Hayot M, Michaud A, Koechlin C, Caron MA, Leblanc P, Prefaut C, et al. Skeletal muscle microbiopsy: a validation study of a minimally invasive technique. Eur Respir J 2005 Mar;25(3):431-40.
[20] Dorph C, Nennesmo I, Lundberg IE. Percutaneous conchotome muscle biopsy. A useful diagnostic and assessment tool. J Rheumatol 2001 Jul;28(7):1591-9.
[21] Henriksson KG. "Semi-open" muscle biopsy technique. A simple outpatient procedure. Acta Neurol Scand 1979 Jun;59(6):317-23.
[22] Poulsen MB, Bojsen-Moller M, Jakobsen J, Andersen H. Percutaneous conchotome biopsy of the deltoid and quadricep muscles in the diagnosis of neuromuscular disorders. J Clin Neuromuscul Dis 2005 Sep;7(1):36-41.
[23] Dietrichson P, Mellgren SI, Skre H. Muscle biopsy with the percutaneous conchotome technique. J Oslo City Hosp 1980 May;30(5):73-9.
[24] Patel H, Syddall HE, Martin HJ, Cooper C, Stewart C, Sayer AA. The feasibility and acceptability of muscle biopsy in epidemiological studies: findings from the Hertfordshire Sarcopenia Study (HSS). J Nutr Health Aging 2011;15(1):10-5.
[25] Lacomis D. The use of percutaneous needle muscle biopsy in the diagnosis of myopathy. Curr Rheumatol Rep 2000 Jun;2(3):225-9.
[26] Magistris MR, Kohler A, Pizzolato G, Morris MA, Baroffio A, Bernheim L, et al. Needle muscle biopsy in the investigation of neuromuscular disorders. Muscle Nerve 1998 Feb;21(2):194-200.
[27] Andonopoulos AP, Papadimitriou C, Melachrinou M, Meimaris N, Vlahanastasi C, Bounas A, et al. Asymptomatic gastrocnemius muscle biopsy: an extremely sensitive and specific test in the pathologic confirmation of sarcoidosis presenting with hilar adenopathy. Clin Exp Rheumatol 2001 Sep;19(5):569-72.
[28] Helliwell TR, Coakley J, Smith PE, Edwards RH. The morphology and morphometry of the normal human tibialis anterior muscle. Neuropathol Appl Neurobiol 1987 Jul;13(4):297-307.
[29] Derry KL, Nicolle MN, Keith-Rokosh JA, Hammond RR. Percutaneous muscle biopsies: review of 900 consecutive cases at London Health Sciences Centre. Can J Neurol Sci 2009 Mar;36(2):201-6.

[30] Evans WJ, Phinney SD, Young VR. Suction applied to a muscle biopsy maximizes sample size. Med Sci Sports Exerc 1982;14(1):101-2.

2

Approach to the Interpretation of Muscle Biopsy

C. Sundaram and Megha S. Uppin
Department of Pathology, Nizam's Institute of Medical Sciences, Hyderabad
India

1. Introduction

The history of muscle biopsy dates back to 1860 when Duchenne first performed a biopsy on a patient with symptoms of myopathy. Introduction of enzyme histochemical methods by Victor Dubowitz in 1970 revolutionised the role of muscle biopsy in the diagnosis of various primary and secondary muscle diseases.[1] Diagnosis of various subtypes of dystrophies was further made easy with beginning of immunohistochemical methods in 1980s. Twenty first century has brought in a new spectacular progress in utility of muscle biopsy with commencement of molecular methods. Significance of muscle biopsy is rising with application of new techniques. The treatment of neuromuscular disorders is also undergoing a parallel and dramatic change with promising genetic therapeutic approaches. Accurate diagnosis of the underlying neuromuscular disease is the need of the day and muscle biopsy forms a gold standard in diagnosis of these diseases.

The indications and techniques of muscle biopsy are discussed in detail in another chapter. Close interaction between pathologist and clinician is necessary for optimal utilization of muscle biopsy sample to get diagnostic information. The muscle biopsy should be planned only after relevant clinical and family history, physical examination findings, laboratory tests including electromyography (EMG), creatine phosphokinase (CPK) and relevant biochemical or serological tests.

2. Site of muscle biopsy

It is necessary to sample a muscle which is clinically involved. This is decided by clinical examination, course of progression of disease and sometimes by imaging studies. It is imperative to biopsy a muscle which is moderately involved. Biopsy from severely affected muscle will only show fat and fibrosis and minimally involved muscle may lack diagnostic histological features. Biopsy has to be taken from muscle belly and avoided from tendon insertion site as it will show central nuclei, variation in fibre size and endomysial fibrosis mimicking myopathy. Muscle site traumatized by EMG needle, sites of recent injections and previous surgery should also be avoided. [2]

In most of the proximal myopathies and generalised/systemic diseases; vastus lateralis is the standard muscle biopsied by international consensus. The site is suitable for biopsy as it is away from major vessels and nerves. [3] The other muscles that are good choices for biopsy are biceps and gastrocnemius. Tibialis anterior is sampled when indicated by imaging studies. Deltoid muscle biopsy is usually avoided as it is a site for injections and may not be involved in all diseases. It is always better to standardize the biopsy from a particular site in the laboratory as the fiber type distribution varies from each site. Biopsies obtained from unusual sites during surgery pose problems for orientation, fiber typing etc.

3. Technique of biopsy

The biopsy can be a needle biopsy or open biopsy. The needle biopsies are dealt within another chapter in detail. Though needle biopsies have largely replaced open biopsies in most parts of the world, certain laboratories still favour open biopsy technique due to feasibility of the procedure and it is usually free of any surgical complications and most importantly because a bigger piece of muscle is available for examination. The sample is kept on a saline soaked gauze piece and transported to the laboratory immediately. It should not be floating in the saline to avoid artefacts.

4. Processing of sample

Orientation of the fibers is of utmost importance since most of the information is provided by transverse sections. The biopsy should be oriented under a dissecting microscope and sample is divided as follows:

1. For electron microscopy, 2-3mm fragments are kept in cacodylate buffered glutaraldehyde and preserved at 4°C.
2. For cryosections, biopsy piece is fresh frozen in isopentane cooled in liquid nitrogen (-170 °C to -180°C) and then sections are cut in cryostat at -18°C to -20°C. These sections are stained with Hematoxylin and Eosin (H&E), Masson trichrome, Modified Gomori's trichrome (MGT). The various enzyme histochemial stains done include myosine adenosine triphosphatase (ATPase) preincubated at P^{H} 9.4, 4.6 and 4.3, succinate dehydrogenase (SDH) and Nicotinamide adenine dinucleotide-Tetrazolium reductase (NADH-TR). Other stains like Per-iodic acid Shiff (PAS), Oil red O, acid phosphatase, cytochrome oxidase, acid maltase and myophosphorylase are done as and when indicated.
3. A part of biopsy is used for routine processing after fixing in buffered formalin
4. For molecular biology, biochemical and genetic analysis, a small tissue is preserved in -80°C. [1,3,4]
5. The fresh unfixed muscle is used for
   a. Detection and quantification of proteins by Gel electrophoresis
   b. Quantification of individual proteins to confirm a deficient or altered protein and provide a precise quantitative measurement by western blot
   c. Demonstrate gene mutations by Polymerase chain reaction (PCR), fluorescent in situ hybridisation (FISH) and others. These techniques are particularly useful in the diagnosis of muscular dystrophies.

The biochemical evaluation of muscle for respiratory enzymes and mitochondria are useful in the evaluation of mitochondrial diseases. These are dealt with in greater detail in other chapters.

5. Normal anatomy

Normal muscle is composed of a number of fascicles which are bound by epimysium and each fascicle in turn is composed of muscle fibers and wrapped by collagen, called perimysium.(Figure 1) The arterioles, nerve bundles, venules and muscle spindles are located in the perimysium. In a child, the muscle fibers are rounded and in an adult, the fibers are polygonal opposed to each other with very little intervening stroma. Myocytes are syncitial and the nuclei are seen subsarcolemmaly. However, 3-4% of internal nuclei are normal. Satellite cells are seen closely applied to the periphery of myofibers. The connective tissue within the fascicle is called endomysium and contains capillary sized blood vessels.

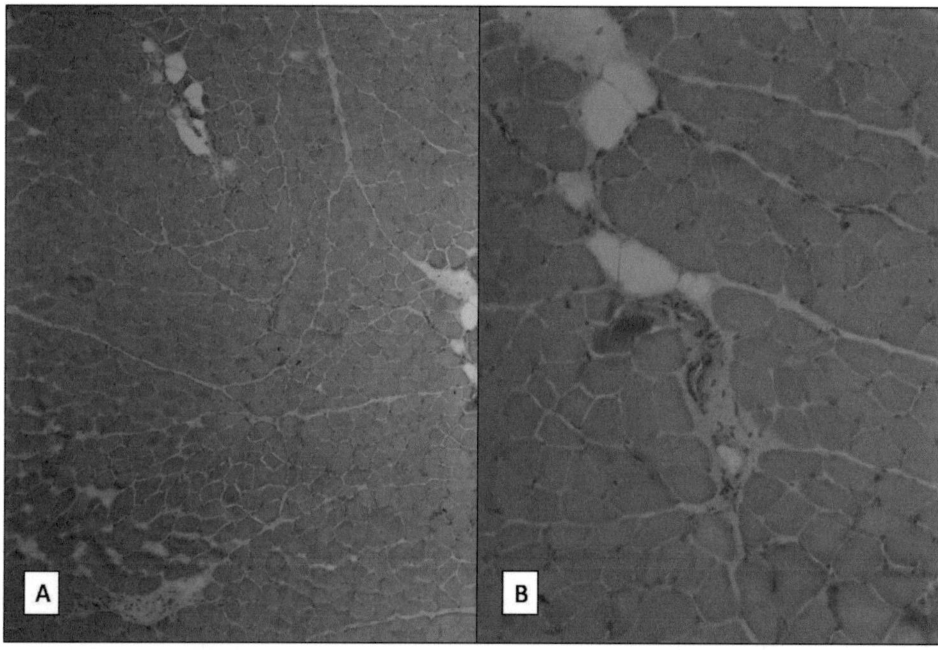

Fig. 1. (A) Fascicular architecture of the muscle with endomysium, perimysium. (H&EX40) (B) The polygonal muscle fibers with subsarcolemmal nuclei (H&EX200)

The interpretation of muscle biopsy will be dealt with according to the type of stain used. The summary of stains and their interpretation is given in Table 1.

Stain	Use
Hematoxylin and Eosin	General architecture and histology
Masson Trichrome	Collagen, fibrosis
Modified Gomori's trichrome	Red ragged fibers, nemaline rods, nuclei, myelinated fibers
Per iodic acid Schiff	Glycogen
Oil red O	Neutral lipid
Acid Phosphatase	Lysosomal enzymes, necrotic fibers
Crystal violet	Amyloid
ATPase PH 9.4	Type 1 fibers pale Type 2 fibers dark
ATP ase 4.6	Type 1 fibers dark Type 2 fibers pale
NADH	Sarcoplasmic structural details
SDH	Oxidative enzyme activity
Cytochrome C Oxidase	Mitochondrial enzyme activity

Table 1. Summary of various stains used in interpretation of muscle biopsy

6. Histochemistry

6.1 Hematoxylin and eosin

This stain helps in evaluation of general architecture of the muscle and variation in the morphology of individual fibers.

H&E is basically used to look at the following changes in muscle:

1. Variation in fascicular architecture
2. Variation in fiber size and shape
3. Necrosis and degeneration of muscle fibers
4. Nuclear characteristics
5. Type and distribution of inflammatory infiltrate
6. Interstitial changes

The architecture of muscle fascicles is assessed on a scanner and the adipose tissue infiltration and fibrosis are noted. The pathological changes if any are noted. Diffuse pattern of involvement is seen in dystrophy, focal in neurogenic and patchy in inflammatory myopathies. Extent of adipose tissue infiltration and fibrosis depend upon the duration of disease and degree of muscle fiber atrophy and contribute to loss of fascicular architecture.

In a normal muscle, there is minimal variation in fiber size which depends on age, gender and muscle. The fiber type variation may be atrophy or hypertrophy and it may selectively involve type 1 or type 2 fibers. The involvement may be diffuse or focal.

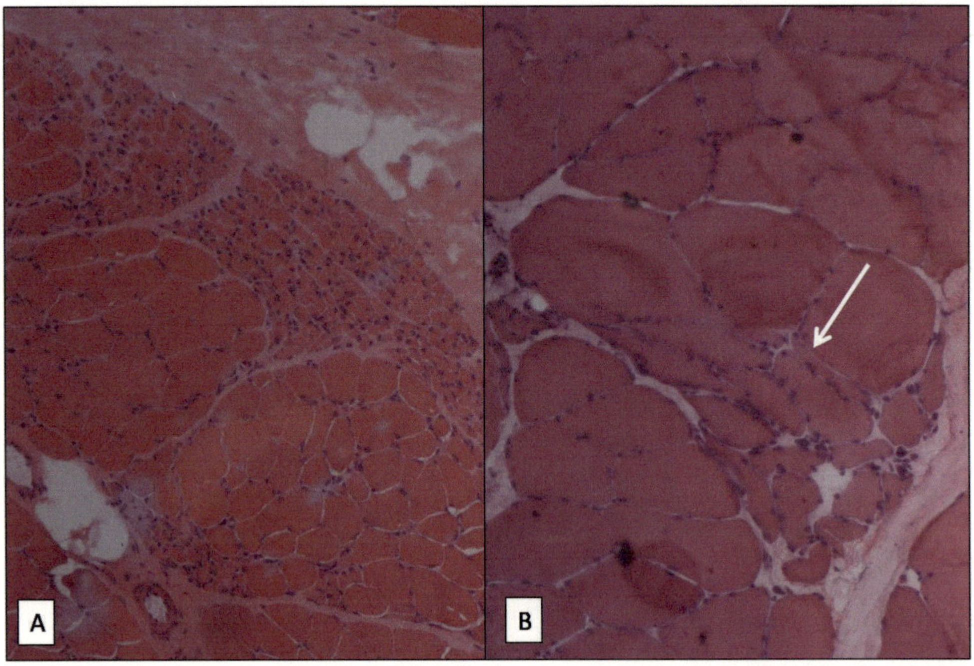

Fig. 2. (A) Large group atrophy H&EX40 (B) Small group atrophy H&EX40 in neurogenic lesions

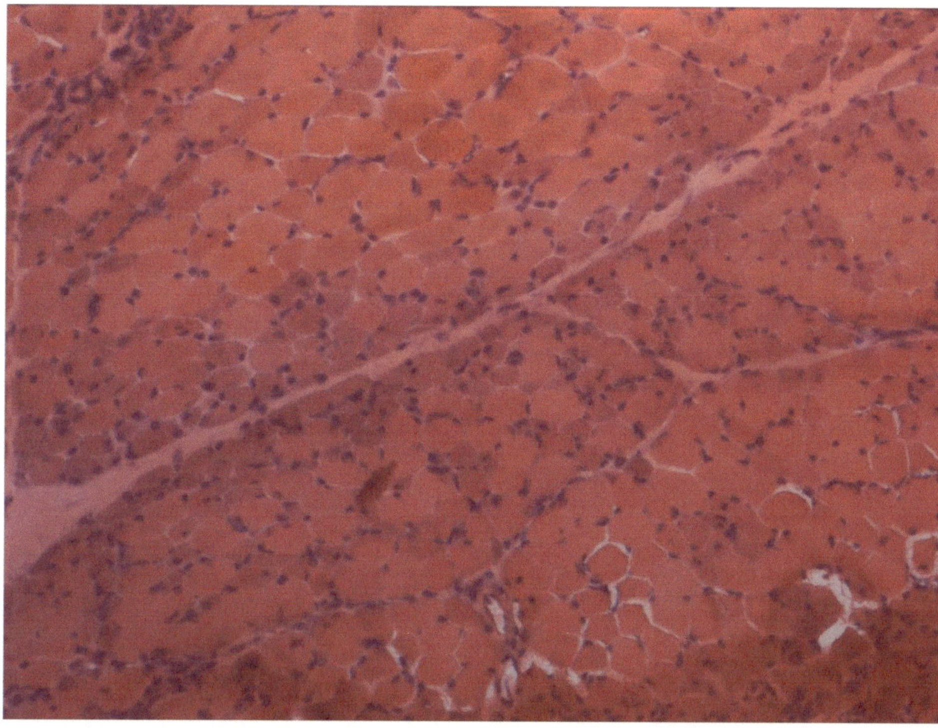

Fig. 3. Perifascicular atrophy in dermatomyositis H&EX40

The atrophic fibers may involve entire fascicle (large group atrophy), small groups of muscle fibers (small group atrophy) or as single fibers. Sometimes all the fibers may be atrophic. These patterns are seen in neurogenic atrophy. (Figure 2) When the atrophic fibers are distributed at the periphery of a fascicle, it is called perifascicular atrophy which is characteristically seen in dermatomyositis, especially juvenile type. (Figure 3) Diffusely distributed atrophic fibers are seen in dystrophies. Atrophy involving selectively type 1 fibers is seen in congenital myopathies, myotonic dystrophy and rheumatoid arthritis.

Fiber hypertrophy is seen in athletes and as compensatory phenomenon in neurogenic atrophies also. They are important findings in dystrophy, especially Limb girdle muscular dystrophy (LGMD). Hypertrophy beyond a particular size leads to splitting. Fiber splitting result in a group of small fibers may be mistaken for small group atrophy. (Figure 4)

6.2 Fiber shape

In normal adult muscle, the muscle fibers are polygonal and in an infant the fibers are rounded. In infants and children there is very little endomysial connective tissue. The fibers become rounded in muscular dystrophies and become angulated and atrophic in denervation.

6.3 Position and number of nuclei

In a normal muscle, nuclei are subsarcolemmal. They are small, oval and dark staining. However, about 3% of fibers in transverse section may show internal nuclei. Large number

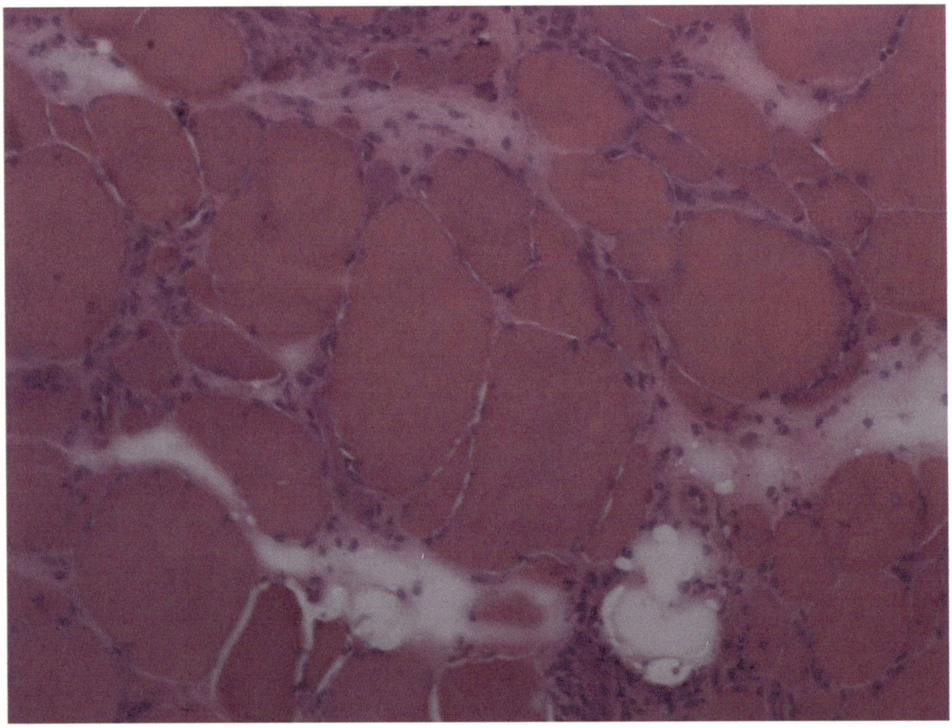

Fig. 4. Split fibers H&EX200

of internal nuclei suggests a myopathy and transverse section is best to assess the same. Dystrophies show about 10-30% internal nuclei and myotonic dystrophy is characterized by profuse number of internal nuclei of about 60%.

Myotubular/centronuclear myopathy shows more than 30% of fibers showing single centrally placed nulei. (Figure 5) Chronic neuropathies like Charcot-Marie-Tooth disease also shows large number of central nuclei. Not only increase in number, the character of nuclei may also vary in various conditions. Vesicular nuclei with prominent nucleoli and transparent nucleoplasm are seen in regenerating fibers, in myopathies and in central nucleus of myotubular/centronuclear myopathy. Tigroid nuclei with granular and clumped chromatin are usually seen in neuropathies and in myotonic dystrophy. Pyknotic nuclei which are dark staining and shrunken are seen in groups with clumping of chromatin. These are seen in neurogenic atrophies and limb girdle dystrophies.

6.4 Necrosis, degeneration and regeneration

A necrotic fiber is pale stained on H&E and infiltrated by phagocytes. This is called myophagocytosis. (Figure 6) This is usually seen in myopathies especially dystrophies like Duchenne muscular dystrophy (DMD). These fibers are highlighted by acid phosphatase and esterase reactions. Sometimes necrotic fibers are seen in inflammatory myopathies, paraneoplastic necrotizing myopathies, after rhabdomyolysis and in acute neuropathies.

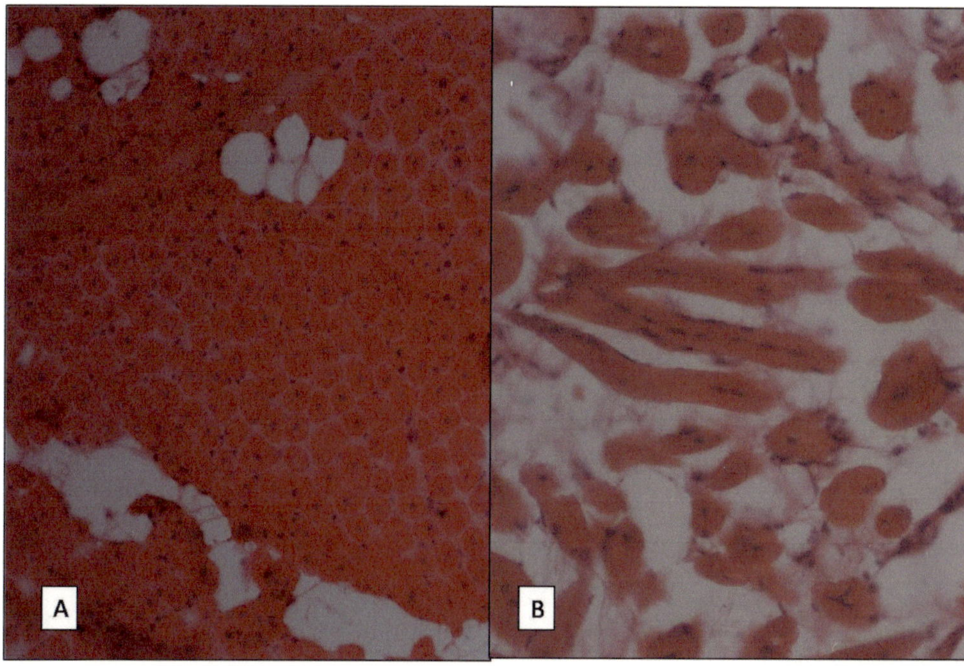

Fig. 5. (A) Muscle fibers showing central nuclei (B) The longitudinal section of the muscle showing central row of nuclei

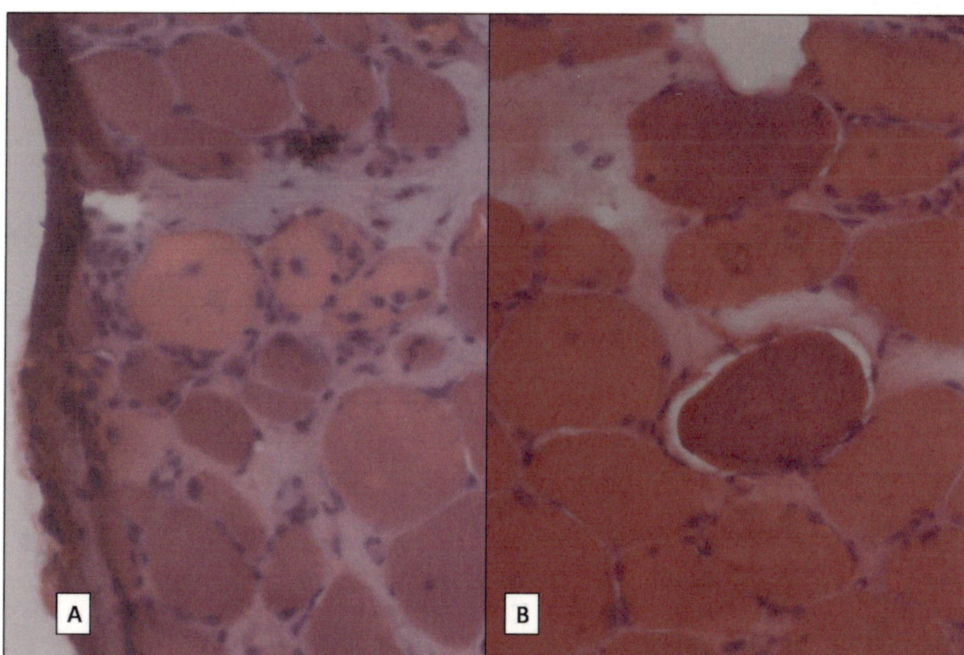

Fig. 6. (A) Myophagocytosis H&EX200 (B) Hyaline fibers H&EX200

A hyalinised fiber is a fiber which has lost its cross striations, has homogenous pale cytoplasm. (Figure 6) Usually these fibers are rounded. They are usually seen in dystrophies. They are highlighted on MGT and Masson trichrome stains.

The granular fiber on H&E shows a coarse granular bluish cytoplasm and represents the ragged red fibers of mitochondrial myopathy on MGT.

Splitting of fibers is seen when a hypertrophic fiber crosses a particular size limit. The nuclei first migrate along the split and large fiber results in a number of small fibers. Fiber splitting is seen normally at tendinous insertion. It is a feature of LGMB and other myopathies and some chronic neuropathies like Charcot-Marie-Tooth disease.

6.5 Interstitial changes

In a normal muscle, the fibers are opposed to each other with very little connective tissue in the endomysium. In muscular dystrophies following myophagocytosis, there is pericellular fibrosis. Fibrosis occurs due to a variety of extracellular matrix proteins and fibrosis occurs in all types of dystrophies, some form of neurogenic atrophies and central core disease also. Adipose tissue infiltrates usually occurs after muscle atrophy. It is more common in DMD but occurs in other dystrophies and late stages of neurogenic atrophies and congenital myopathies. The degree of fibrosis is well brought out by Masson trichrome stain. (Figure 7)

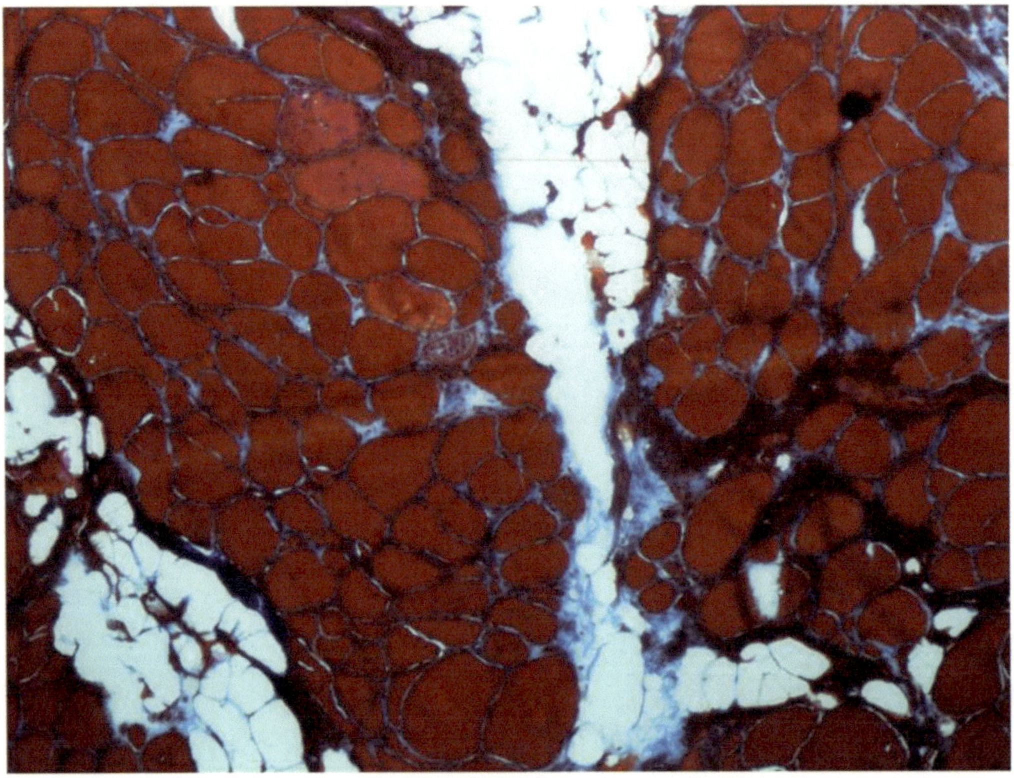

Fig. 7. Pericellular fibrosis highlighted by Masson trichrome. MTX100

6.6 Inflammatory cell infiltrates

Normal muscle is devoid of any inflammatory cells. Cellular infiltrates are seen in inflammatory myopathies like dermatomyositis, inclusion body myositis (IBM). (Figure 8) Necrotic muscle fibers are invaded by mononuclear cells which are seen in almost all dystrophies. Inflammatory cells can occur in toxic, necrotizing and dystrophic muscle diseases especially fasioscapulohumeral dystrophy (FSHD), DMD, dysferlinopathy and other LGMDs apart from inflammatory myopathies.

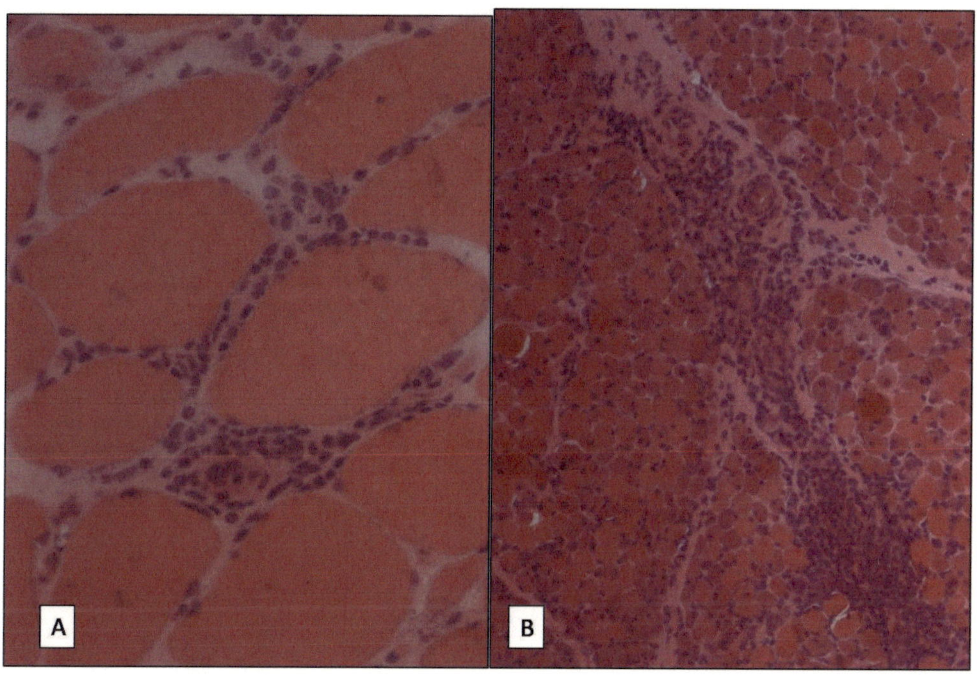

Fig. 8. (A) Inflammation around non necrotic fibers in IBM H&EX40 (B) Perivascular inflammation in dermatomyositis. H&EX40

The infiltrate is composed of B ells, CD4 positive cells and dendritic cells in dermatomyositis; CD 8 positive cells, dendritic cells and macrophages in polymyositis and IBM which can be demonstrated by immunohistochemistry.

The modified Gomori's trichrome (MGT) stain is useful to stain the red ragged fibers; the hallmark of mitochondrial myopathy. (Figure 9) Red ragged fibers are also seen in other conditions like dystrophies (LGMD), dermatomyositis, older individuals and Zidovudine associated myopathy in HIV patients. [5,6]

Tubular aggregates and cytoplasmic bodies are nonspecific and are seen with MGT as red. (Figure 10) Tubular aggregates are seen in periodic paralysis, dysferlinopathy, exertional myalgia etc. Cytoplasmic bodies are seen in collagen vascular disease, IBM and others.

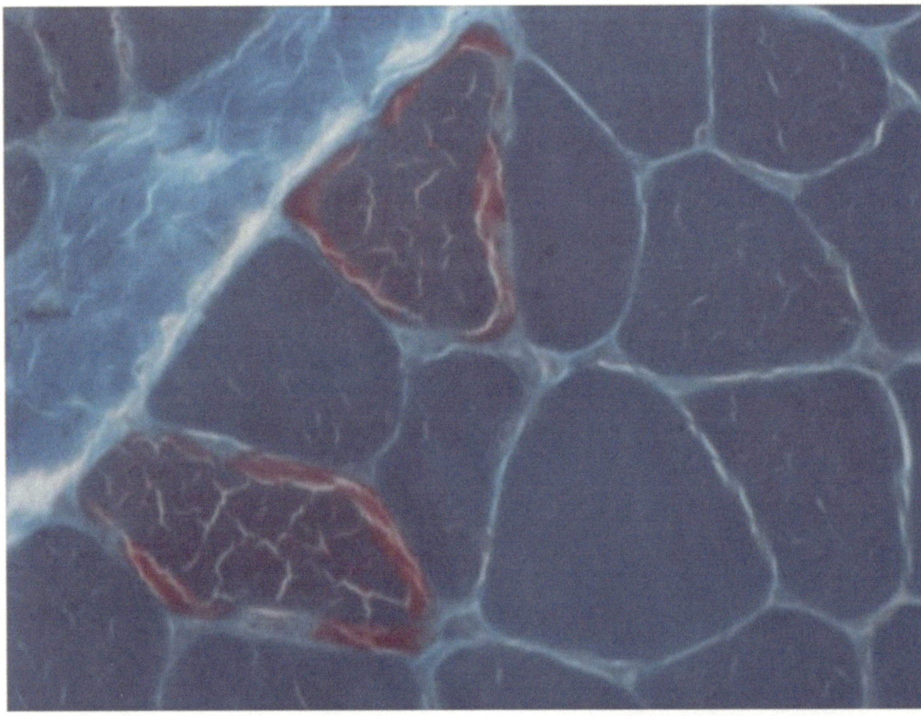

Fig. 9. Red ragged fibers of mitochondrial myopathy MGTX200

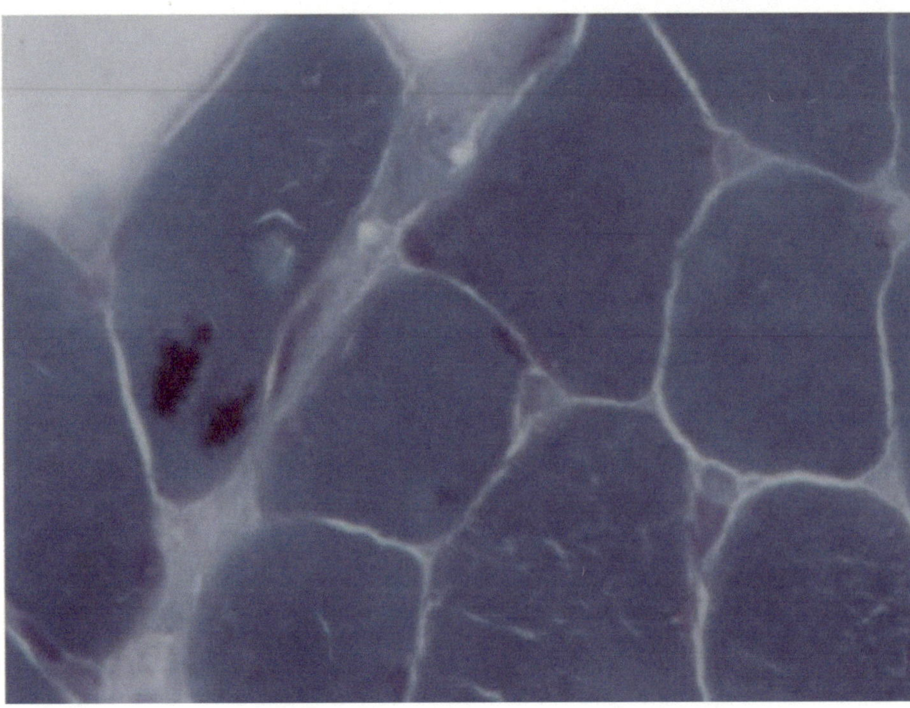

Fig. 10. Tubulofilamentous inclusions MGTX400

Rod bodies characteristically stain red with MGT.(Figure 11) The rods are delicate and accumulate subsarcolemmaly. They stain negative with ATPase, NADH and SDH as they lack myosin and mitochondria. Rods are characteristic of nemaline myopathy but also seen in central core disease and various other diseases which include neurogenic disorders (amyotrophic lateral sclerosis, spinal muscular atrophy, undefined), inflammatory myopathies (dermatomyositis, polymyositis, periarteritis nodosa), metabolic myopathy (mitochondrial myopathy), muscular dystrophy (LGMD) and some undefined myopathies. [7]

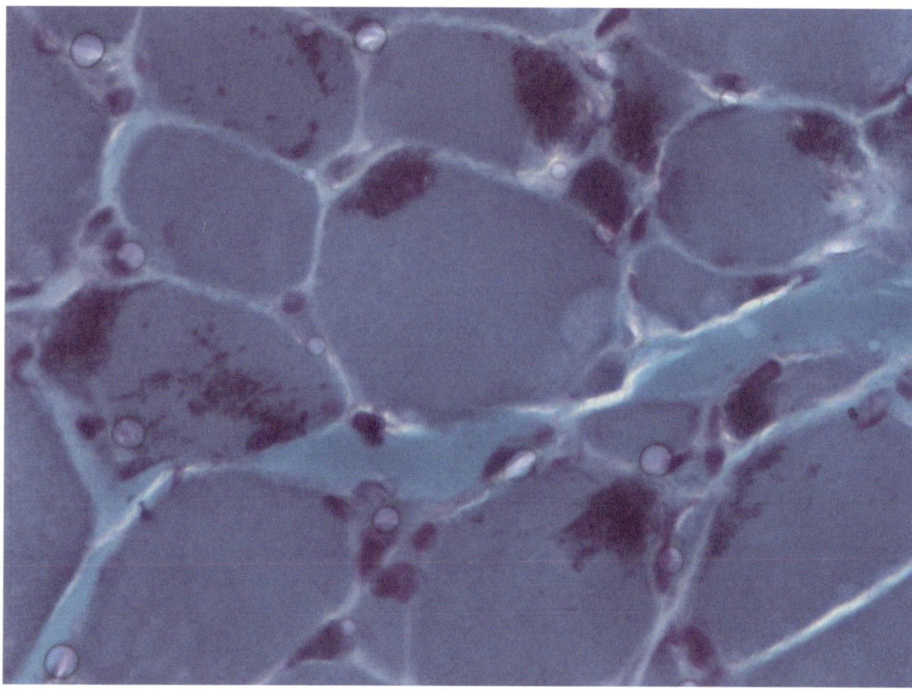

Fig. 11. Rod bodies seen in subsarcolemmal and perinuclear position in a case of nemaline myopathy. MGTX400

MGT also stains nuclei and myelinated fibers.

The per-iodic-acid Schiff (PAS) and Oil red O demonstrate glycogen and neutral lipid respectively. (Figure 12) These two stains are useful for metabolic myopathies. Acid phosphatase identifies lysosomal enzymes and hence identifies necrotic fibers. Masson trichrome is useful to demonstrate fibrosis and fibrinoid necrosis. Congo red and crystal violet stains demonstrate amyloid.

Vacuoles

Vacuoles are of two types- one type contains some material within and the other appears as just empty spaces. The former are called as rimmed vacuoles and on H&E they contain basophilic granular material and on MGT they appear as having red granules.(Figure 13) They appear in number of conditions like IBM, distal myopathies, oculopharyngeal muscular dystrophies, myofibrillar myopathies and others. In glycogen storage disease, vacuoles appear on H&E. The vacuoles are seen in acid maltase deficiency of childhood (Pompe's disease) and adulthood (McArdle's disease) and Glycogenses V.

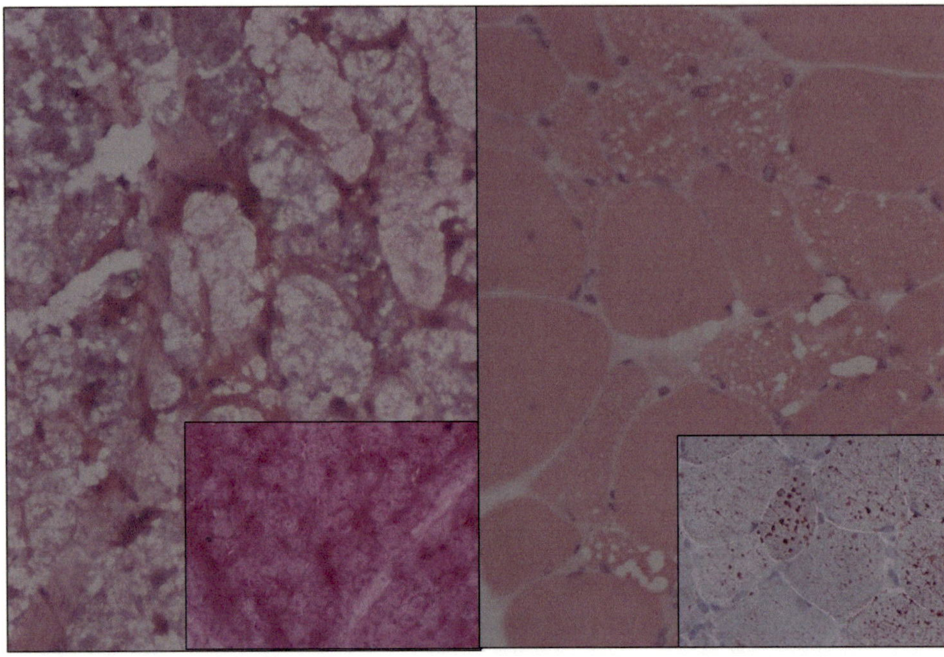

Fig. 12. (A) Vacuolated cytoplasm in glycogen storage disease.H&EX100.Inset: Intracellular glycogen content. PASX200 (B) Small vacuoles in the sarcoplasm of muscle fibers in lipid storage myopathy. Inset: lipid droplets stained red by Oil Red O. Oil Red OX200

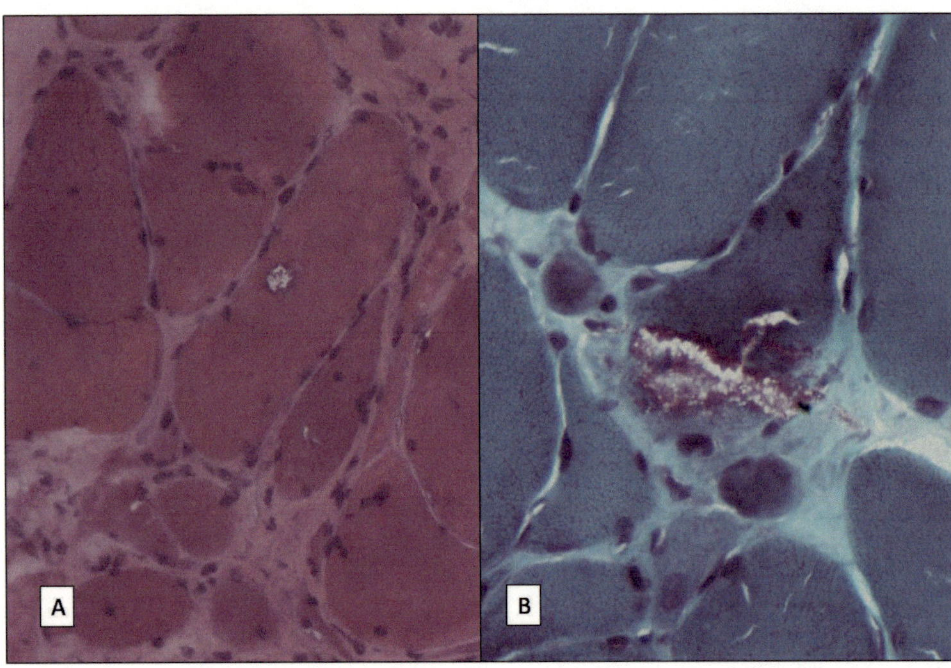

Fig. 13. (A) Rimmed vacuoles showing basophilic rimming. H&EX200 (B) Rimmed vacuoles showing red granular rimming. MGTX400

The diagnosis can be established by demonstrating absence of acid maltase and phoshphorylase respectively. Excess glycogen accumulation in vacuoles and in the fibers can be demonstrated by PAS stain in glycogenoses. Similarly, lipid accumulation is demonstrated in vacuoles or in the fibers in carnitine deficiency or in disorders of mitochondrial beta oxidation. They show cytochrome C oxidase enzyme deficiency.

7. Enzyme histochemistry

ATPase: In myosine ATPase preincubated at PH 9.4, type 1 fibers are pale and type 2 fibers are dark. At PH 4.6 and 4.3, the reaction is reversed and type 1 fibers are dark and type 2a and 2b fibers are light with variable intensity. Owing to these staining characteristics on ATPase, this stain is used to demonstrate abnormalities in fiber types and distribution of the two types of fibers. (Figure 14)

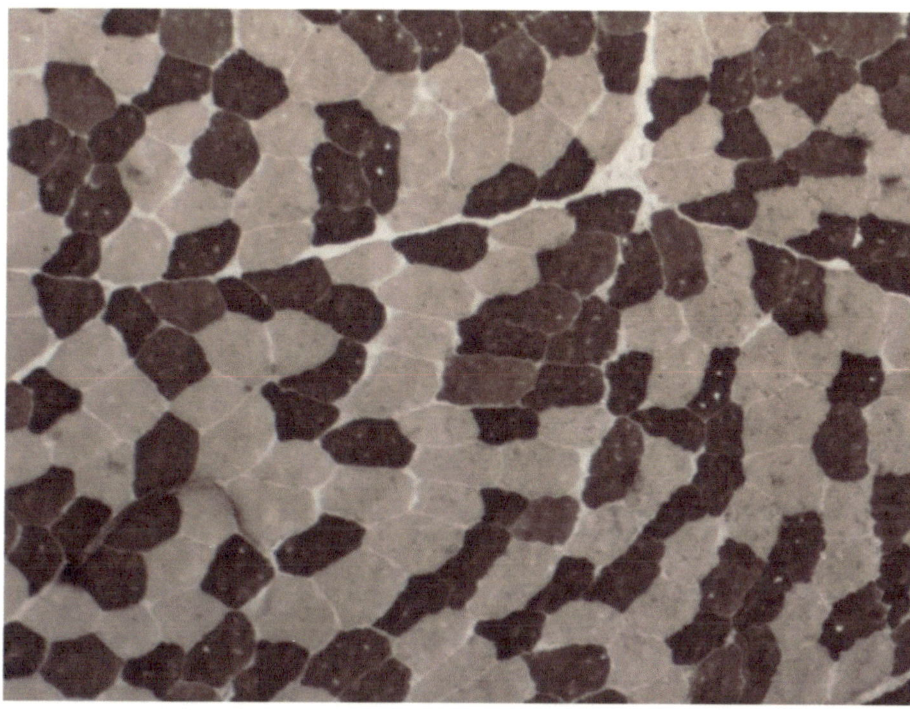

Fig. 14. ATPase at PH 9.4 showing checkerboard pattern with pale Type 1 fibers and dark Type 2 fibers. ATPX100

In muscles like vastus lateralis, type 1, 2a and 2b are one third each. Type 1 and 2 fibers are intermixed in a checkerboard pattern. Type 1 fibers of more than 55% is said to be type 1 predominance and similarly type 2A and type 2B each of 55% constitute predominance of that fiber subtype. Type 2 predominance is called when type 2 fibers are more than 80%.

Type 1 predominance indicates a myopathy; either dystrophy or congenital myopathy whereas type 2 predominance in motor neuron disease.

Type I predominance is normally seen in gastrocnemius and deltoid and hence caution should be exercised in interpreting biopsies from these sites.

In addition to type predominance, fiber type grouping which is characteristic of neurogenic lesions is also best assessed on ATPase stain.

Atrophy of particular type of fibers is also evaluated by ATPase. Selective type 1 fiber atrophy is seen in congenital myopathies and myotonic dystrophy. Selective type 2 atrophy is common and is seen in many conditions. These include steroid myopathy, disuse, polymyalgia rheumatica, collagen vascular diseases, pyramidal tract disease, mental retardation, myasthenia gravis etc. [1,2] Type 2 atrophy usually involves type 2B or both type 2A and type 2B; however only type 2A atrophy is uncommon. [1]

Fiber specific hypertrophy is very uncommon.

Subtle changes in fiber size are best made out by plotting histograms. [1]

SDH and NADH

These enzyme histochemical stains bring about various structural abnormalities of muscle fibers and being oxidative enzymes are important in diagnosis of mitochondrial myopathies.

The abnormal fibers of mitochondrial myopathy are seen as "blue ragged fibers "on SDH and NADH and they are the counterpart of red ragged fibers on MGT. (Figure 15) COX is a mitochondrial enzyme and its activity is absent in mitochondrial myopathy or abnormalities. A combination of COX-SDH brings about more number of abnormal fibers in mitochondrial myopathy. [8]

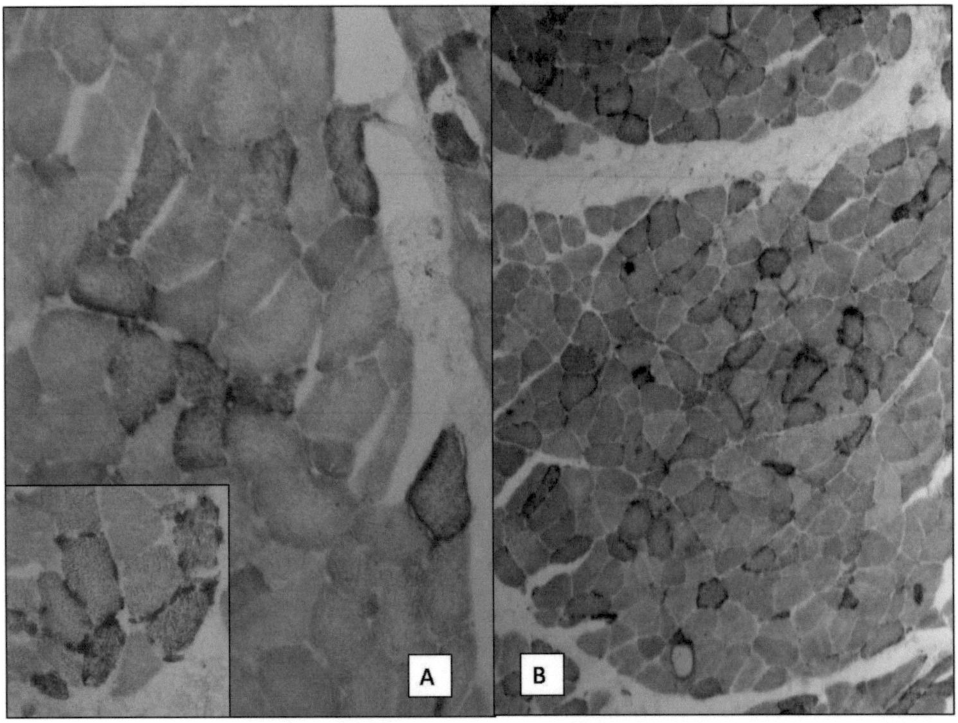

Fig. 15. (A) Blue ragged fibers of mitochondrial myopathy. SDHX100 Inset: The same fibers on higher magnification. SDHX400 (B) The same muscle showing more abnormal fibers on COX-SDHX40

NADH-TR highlights the sarcoplasmic reticulum and oxidative enzyme activity, Structural abnormalities like cores, targets, whorles, lobulated fibers are best seen on NADH-TR. SDH is an oxidative enzyme and mitochondrial abnormalities are highlighted by SDH. Cores and lobulated fibers are also seen on SDH.(Figure 16) Acid maltase, myophsprylase are done as and when indicated clinically (glycogen storage diseases).The myofibrillar abnormalities include central/minicores, target, targetoid fibers, ring fibers, whorled fibers and lobulated fibers.

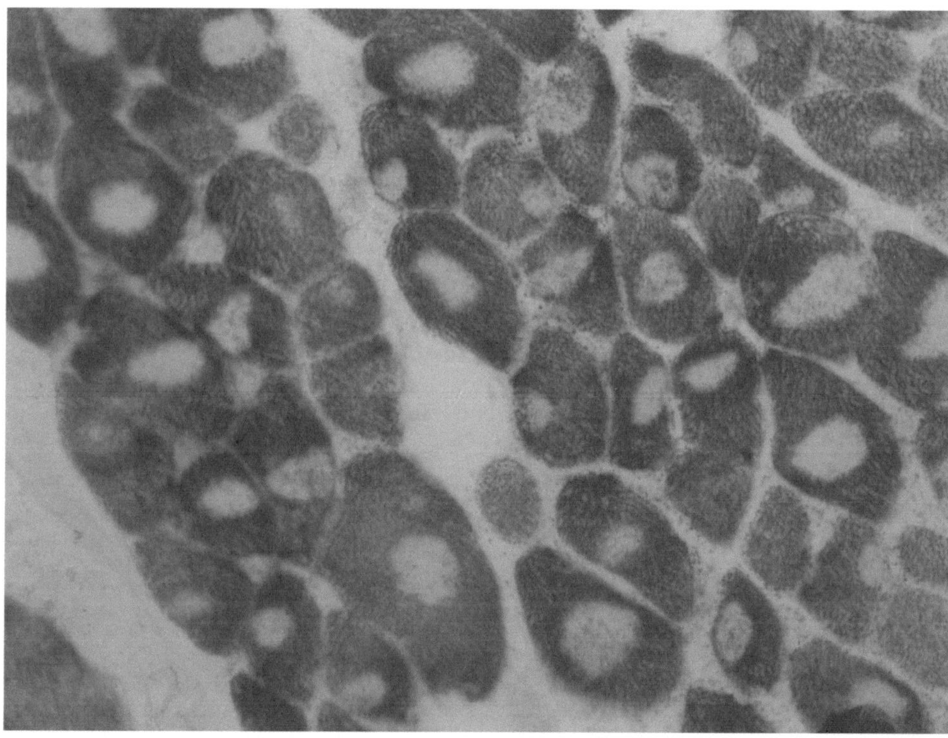

Fig. 16. Central cores in a case of central core disease. SDHX100

Central cores are seen as pale areas of staining on oxidative enzyme staining like NADH and SDH. The cores are usually single and central but may be eccentric and multiple. They are not seen on H&E, ATPase, MGT but seen on phosphorylase. The rim of the core is devoid of mitochondria and hence lacks oxidative enzyme activity. Central cores are seen usually in type 1 fibers. Central cores are seen in many fibers in central core disease. Central cores are not limited to central core disease as they are seen in hypertrophic cardiomyopathy associated with missense mutations in the beta myosine heavy chain gene, MHY7 [9], autosomal dominant myopathy associated with ACTA 1 gene mutations. [10] Multiple minicores seen on oxidative enzyme reactions both in transverse and longitudinal sections are seen in multiminicore disease (MmD) and it is a histopathologic continuum with central core disease. Many cases of MmD are caused by recessive mutations in the selenoprotein NI (SENPI) gene [11] and same due to recessive RYR1 mutations. [12,13]

Target fibers are characterised by three distinct zones where central zone is devoid of oxidative enzyme activity, middle zone of intense activity and outer zone of intermediate activity. They are usually seen in type 1 fibers when the three zones are not clearly demarcated, the target fibers resemble central cores and they are called targetoid fibers. Target fibers are a feature of chronic neuropathies.

Moth eaten fibers show irregular disruption of myofibrillar network. These are seen on NADH or SDH and may be mistaken for minicores or cores. Moth eaten fibers are seen in dystrophies including LGMD, congenital muscular dystrophy and various myopathies including dermatomyositis. (Figure 17)

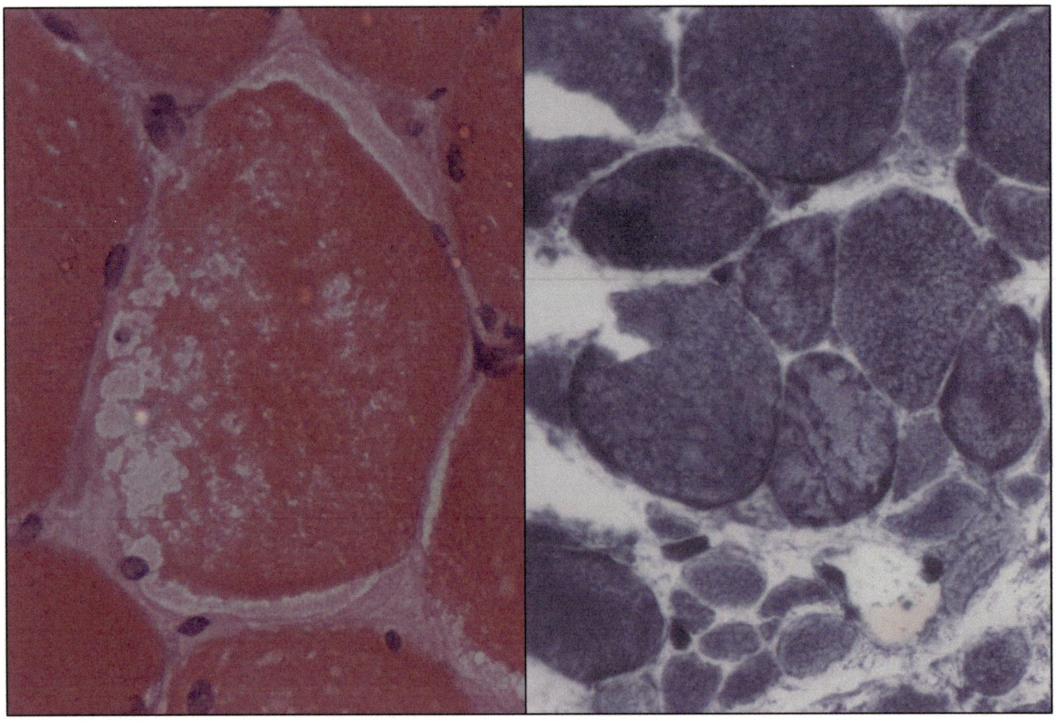

Fig. 17. (Left) Moth eaten fiber on H&E X400 and (Right) on SDHX200

Ring fibers and whorled/coiled fibers are due to various patterns of disarray of myofibrils. They are seen in various dystrophies. (Figure 18) Ring fibers are seen in myotonic dystrophy whereas whored fibers are seen in LGMD and chronic neuropathies.

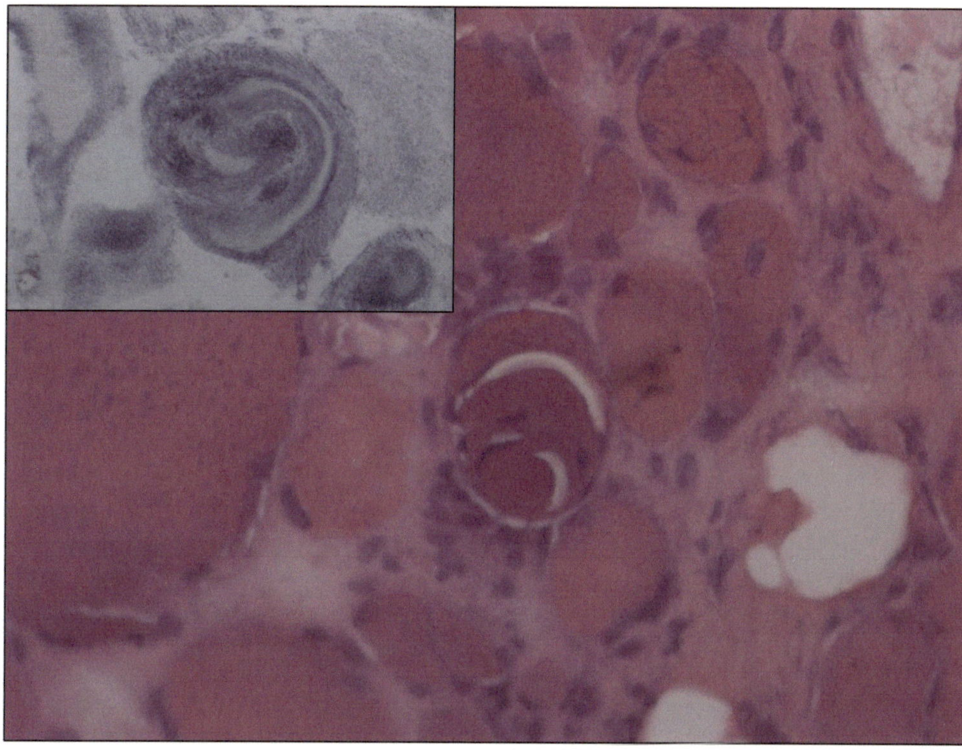

Fig. 18. Whorled fibers in a case of limb girdle muscular dystrophy H&EX200. Inset: The same fiber on SDHX400

Lobulated fibers show intense oxidative enzyme activity at the periphery of the fiber and usually involve type 1 fibers. They are nonspecific and are seen in many conditions which include LGMD particularly calpainopathy, congenital muscular dystrophy, mitochondrial myopathy and others.

8. Conclusion

Muscle biopsy is essential for accurate diagnosis and treatment. Optimal utilization of the sample with appropriate stains and study of the pathologic features is important for making a diagnosis. Accurate interpretation of muscle biopsy guides appropriate immunohistochemical and molecular genetic studies.

9. References

[1] Dubowitz C, Sewry CA. In: Dubowitz C, Sewry CA (eds.) Muscle biopsy. A practical approach. Philadelphia, USA: Elsevier, Saunders, 2007.

[2] Engel WK. Focal myopathic changes produced by electromyographic and hypodermic needles. Archives of Neurology (Chicago). 1967;16:509-11

[3] Kakulas BA, Adams RD. Diseases of muscle. Pathological foundations of clinical myology. 4th ed. Philadelphia: Harper and Row, 1985.

[4] Harriman DGF. Diseases of Muscle. In: Adams JH, Corsellis JAN, Duchen LW, eds. Greenfield's neuropathology. 4th ed. Edward Arnold, 1984: 1026-96.

[5] Schoffner Jm, Lott Mt, Lezza Ams, Seibel P., Ballinger Sw, Wallace Dc. Myoclonic epilepsy and ragged-red fiber disease (MERRF) is associated with a mitochondrial DNA tRNAlys mutation. Cell 1990; 61: 931-37

[6] Arnaudo E; Dalakas MC; Shanske S; Moraes CT; Di Mauro S; Schon EA. Depletion of muscle mitochondrial DNA in AIDS patients with zidovudine-induced myopathy. Lancet 1991;337:508-10.

[7] Shoei-Show Liou, Shun-Sheng Chen, Itsuro Higuchi, Hidetoshi Fukunaga, Mitsuhiro Osame. Diagnostic role of nemaline rod in neuromuscular disease. Acta Neurol Sinica 1992;1: 218-23.

[8] Fananapazir L, Dalakas MC, Cyran F, Cohn G, Epstein ND. Missense mutations in the beta-myosin heavy-chain gene cause central core disease in hypertrophic cardiomyopathy. Proc Natl Acad Scie U S A. 1993;90:3993-7.

[9] Kaindl AM, Rüschendorf F, Krause S, Goebel HH, Koehler K, Becker C, Pongratz D, Müller-Höcker J, Nürnberg P, Stoltenburg-Didinger G, Lochmüller H, Huebner A. Missense mutations of ACTA1 cause dominant congenital myopathy with cores. J Med Genet. 2004;41:842-8.

[10] Ferreiro A, Fardeau M. 80th ENMC International workshop on muti-minicore disease:1st International MmD workshop. 12-13 May 2000, Soestduinen, The Netherlands. Neuromuscular Disorders 2002;12:60-8.

[11] Monnier N, Ferreiro A, Marty I et al. A homozygous splicing mutation causing depletion of skeletal muscle RYR1 is associated with multi-minicore disease congenital myopathy with opthalmoplegia. Human Molecular Genetics. 2003;12:1171-78.

[12] Jungbluth H, Muller CR, Halliger-Keller B et al. Autosomal recessive inheritance of RYR1 mutations in a congenital myopathy with cores. Neurology 2002;59:284-7.

Part 2

Muscle Biopsy: Biomedical Research

3

Generation and Use of Cultured Human Primary Myotubes

Lauren Cornall, Deanne Hryciw,
Michael Mathai and Andrew McAinch
Victoria University
Australia

1. Introduction

Cell culture is a widely used technique in biomedical research. It permits the analysis of cell specific functions which can relate to changes in certain disease states at the single cell level. A number of cell culture models have been established. These include immortalised cell lines which replicate indefinitely in culture and retain the ability to differentiate and primary cell lines which can be isolated directly from the host tissue and grown in culture. However, primary cell lines have limited replicative potential and become senescent in culture. In the case of muscle cells, cell lines can provide a valuable means of investigating physiology in the absence of confounding factors (such as circulating hormones, adipokines and other bioactive molecules) which arise when dealing with the body as a whole.

Human primary cell lines provide additional benefits in research, when compared to immortalised cell lines, as primary cultures have been shown to retain the metabolic characteristics of the tissue donor and thus reflect alterations in metabolism as seen in specific disease states such as obesity and type 2 diabetes mellitus (Gaster et al., 2004; Steinberg et al., 2006). Of particular interest to the treatment of myopathies is the use of human primary myotube cultures which can be isolated from muscle extracts in normal and diseased states. We (Chen et al., 2005; McAinch et al., 2006b; McAinch et al., 2007; Steinberg et al., 2006) and others (Bell et al., 2010; Mott et al., 2000; Thompson et al., 1996) have shown that the resultant myotube cultures retain phenotypic traits of the donor related to defects in fatty acid oxidation, impairment of insulin stimulated glucose uptake, leptin and/or adiponectin resistance. Thus, there is increased clinical relevance associated with the use of primary cell cultures in researching disease pathogenesis, making human primary cell cultures an invaluable tool in assessing aberrant cellular metabolism and how this may be targeted experimentally to alleviate metabolic dysregulation.

In this chapter we aim to provide the reader with a detailed explanation of the methodological considerations in isolating and culturing of human primary myotubes and their subsequent experimental uses.

2. Current applications of human primary myotubes

2.1 Skeletal muscle cell culture

The skeletal muscle is a highly metabolically active tissue and has a profound influence over systemic metabolic function through the regulation of carbohydrate and fatty acid metabolism (Baron et al., 1988; Zurlo et al., 1990). Historically, the study of cellular mechanisms regulating skeletal muscle physiology was limited by difficulties in maintaining metabolically viable isolated muscle extracts and the ability to manipulate specific variables *in vivo*. The development of cell culture models has provided an invaluable tool by which cellular physiology can be studied. Over the last several decades cell culture techniques have evolved and the resultant studies have contributed greatly to the current understanding of cellular metabolism. A vast number of cell types are cultured to investigate pertinent research questions. Typically the cells used in these models will either be an immortalised cell line or a primary cell line, each of which has distinct advantages. Herein, we provide a brief discussion of the development of both immortalised and primary skeletal muscle cell culture models.

2.1.1 Immortalised cell lines

Undifferentiated immortalised skeletal muscle cell lines have an indefinite myogenic potential, with cells continuing to undergo mitotic divisions when maintained in the appropriate culture conditions. Accordingly, these cell lines expand rapidly in culture to provide a readily repeatable experimental model and can provide an alternative to isolating primary cell lines. A key consideration with the use of immortalised cell lines is the retention of physiological functions similar to that of the tissue source (Obinata, 2001). Therefore it is important that immortalised cell lines are adequately characterised to demonstrate that differentiated cell lines recapitulate the physiology of the original tissue.

Clonal cell lines were initially derived from transgenic animal models, tumour cells, treatment of cells with carcinogens or arose through mutations of specific cells within primary cultures (Efrat et al., 1988; Obinata, 2001; Richler & Yaffe, 1970; Todaro & Green, 1963; Todaro et al., 1963). These cells do not readily respond to the normal apopotic signals and continue to replicate and divide beyond the life span of un-mutated cells. Isolation and cloning of these myogenic cells enables clonal cell lines to be formed. Despite their benefits in experimental molecular and cellular biology, the relative lack of clonal cell lines and the difficulty in generating new cell lines has inhibited research capacity. More recent techniques utilised to produce immortalised cell lines involve cellular transfection with immortalising genes or oncogenes (Condon et al., 2002; Douillard-Guilloux et al., 2009; Jat et al., 1991). Such methods utilise transfection of genes including telomerase, SV40 Large T-antigen, cyclin-dependent kinase 4 and Bmi to induce immortalisation of a number of cell types (Condon et al., 2002; Di Donna et al., 2003; Douillard-Guilloux et al., 2009). These methods are limited initially by the number of cells stably expressing the transfected DNA needed to generate a viable population of the immortalised cell line. Additionally, cellular incorporation of the immortalising gene can occur at different sites in theoretically identical cells which can lead to variable gene expression and cellular behaviours. The use of clonal cell lines is further confounded by the potential for the introduced DNA to alter the cellular phenotype and therefore cellular physiology (Ridley et al., 1988). This issue may also be apparent in certain cell lines derived from transgenic animal models and tumour cells which reflect the host's expression of certain genes and proteins (Efrat et al., 1988). This may be partially overcome by the generation of conditionally immortalised cell lines in which the effect of the immortalising agent is abrogated under certain culture conditions, such as changes in serum concentrations or temperature (Macpherson et al., 2004; Obinata, 2001).

Immortalised cell lines that are commonly used for investigating skeletal muscle physiology are L6 and C_2C_{12} skeletal muscle myotubes which are derived from rat and mouse origin, respectively (Blau et al., 1985; Yaffe, 1968; Yaffe & Saxel, 1977). These cell lines can be terminally differentiated into skeletal muscle myotubes by altering the culture environment to low serum conditions and thus provide a relevant method of investigating muscle physiology.

The L6 cell line was initially described by Yaffe (1968). This cell line was established from newborn rat thigh muscle treated with the carcinogen 20(3) methylcholanthrene in the growth medium during the first two growth passages (Yaffe, 1968). In initial experiments, the L6 cell line was maintained *in vitro* for more than 18 months without losing the ability to fuse to form differentiated myotubes (Yaffe, 1968). In subsequent studies, Richler & Yaffe (1970) observed the L6 cell line to develop into multinucleate, cross-striated myotubes which retain contractile properties. The clonal mouse C_2C_{12} cell line is a diploid sub-clone generated by Blau et al., (1985) as a derivative of the cell line described by Yaffe & Saxel (1977). This cell line was developed by Yaffe & Saxel (1977) from thigh muscle of CH3 mice and was shown to retain the capacity to proliferate and differentiate in culture. The C_2C_{12} cell line has subsequently been used in muscle physiology studies due to its rapid proliferation and ability to differentiate to form contractile myotubes which express myogenic proteins (Blau et al., 1985; Yaffe & Saxel, 1977). The initial characterisation of both the L6 and C_2C_{12} cell lines indicating pronounced differentiation and retention of contractile properties suggest that these cell lines are appropriate models for studying muscle physiology.

2.1.2 Primary cell lines

Adult myotubes are not capable of mitotic divisions and therefore primary skeletal muscle culture systems rely on the ability to induce activation and subsequent myogenic differentiation of quiescent satellite cells from within the muscle fibre (Berggren et al., 2007; Blau & Webster, 1981). Unlike immortalised cell lines, once isolated, primary skeletal muscle cultures are fated for senescence and cease to proliferate after a relatively short period in culture. Consistent with this Machida et al., (2004) showed that with passaging the myogenic potential (as measured by myogenic markers, proliferation and differentiation potential) of rat primary cells to decrease. However primary cells do retain phenotypic traits of the donor cells, and are able to be cultured from small muscle samples of approximately 50 mg to counter this limitation (Berggren et al., 2007; McAinch et al., 2007). For example, studies investigating the phenotype of human primary skeletal muscle myotubes have shown the retention of aberrant glucose metabolism in primary myotubes cultured from insulin resistant Pima Indians (Thompson et al., 1996). Further studies have demonstrated that phenotypic traits of impaired insulin signalling (Bell et al., 2010), fatty acid uptake and oxidation (Bell et al., 2010; Mott et al., 2000), action of the anti -obesogenic and -diabetic adipokines, adiponectin and leptin and aberrant expression of genes which regulate substrate metabolism within skeletal muscle (McAinch & Cameron-Smith, 2009; McAinch et al., 2006b; McAinch et al., 2007) are also retained. Thus, cultured primary myotubes enable the study of muscle cell structure and function in any number of physiological and pathophysiological states. Moreover, cultured myotubes enable the investigation of many metabolic abnormalities that exist *in vivo*, while eliminating confounding environmental influences on the muscle (such as circulating hormones, adipokines and other bioactive factors). Myogenic satellite cells can be isolated from a number of tissues including skeletal muscle (Blau & Webster, 1981; Chen et al., 2005; Gaster et al., 2001a; McAinch & Cameron-Smith, 2009). When cultured in specific conditions, quiescent satellite cells isolated from donor skeletal muscle can be stimulated to re-enter the cell cycle and proliferate before being terminally differentiated to recapitulate the phenotype of skeletal muscle from the donor.

As such primary skeletal muscle myotubes have multiple research applications including but not limited to; 1) the study of the effects of myopathies and systemic metabolic diseases on skeletal muscle function, 2) tissue regeneration and renewal for tissue engineering purposes, 3) gene therapy and 4) drug screening (Berggren et al., 2007; Chen et al., 2005; Kessler et al., 1996; Loro et al., 2010; McAinch & Cameron-Smith, 2009; McAinch et al., 2006a; McAinch et al., 2006b; McAinch et al., 2007; Stern-Straeter et al., 2008).

The following sections outline the process of culturing human primary myotubes from their isolation from muscle biopsies to their growth and maintenance in culture and finally a brief look at their current and future applications. At this point we are compelled to mention that methodological variations arise at almost every stage of primary myotube culture, especially in regards to medium composition and the differentiation protocol. Whilst we endeavour to consider the differences in protocols and the implications of these, we primarily report the established methods of our laboratory. Therefore some optimisation may be necessary on behalf of the end user where experimental outcomes differ significantly.

3. The muscle biopsy

A number of techniques can be used to obtain a skeletal muscle biopsy including needle biopsy and surgical excision (Dietrichson et al., 1987; Tarnopolsky et al., 2011). Successful isolation of myogenic satellite cells can be undertaken from small samples of muscle biopsies ranging in size from 50-100 mg (wet weight) (McAinch et al., 2007). This suggests that the typical muscle yield from suction-enhanced needle biopsies is sufficient to culture viable primary myotubes (Melendez et al., 2007; Tarnopolsky et al., 2011). The use of needle biopsy has additional benefits in the relative ease of obtaining muscle biopsies, enabling sampling from a number of accessible skeletal muscles with only the use of local anaesthetic (Dietrichson et al., 1987). The suction-enhanced method described by Tarnopolsky et al., (2011) is described briefly as follows.

The area from which the muscle biopsy is to be obtained is sterilised and the skin and subcutaneous tissue is numbed with a local anaesthetic. A small stab incision (4-5 mm) is made in the skin at the biopsy site. With the aperture closed, the biopsy needle is advanced through this incision to penetrate at least 1 cm beyond the fascia. This motion will be associated with the sensation of deep pressure within the muscle. Once the needle is in position within the muscle, the aperture is opened, and if using a suction enhanced technique, suction is applied using a sterile 60 ml syringe (approximately 20 ml per sample). It is important to note that the equipment used by these authors is modified to accommodate the suction procedure. However, the biopsy size is significantly increased by using suction compared to no suction (approximately 125 mg compared to 35 mg, respectively. However significant variation in muscle biopsy size exists). The needle is then closed to isolate the muscle biopsy. The needle can then be rotated to obtain another muscle sample as above. The authors describe taking up to 3 samples in quick succession in the one biopsy to obtain adequate muscle sample and is associated with minimum discomfort. The needle is removed using a twisting motion during withdrawal. Pressure is applied to the skin incision and it is closed with a single suture or a tape closure (although a suture may be associated with a lesser degree of scarring) and then pressure is reapplied for 10-15 minutes often with concomitant icing. It is then important the area be kept clean by the subject in the period following the procedure. If closed with a suture, the suture is removed 6 days after the biopsy procedure.

Alternately, skeletal muscle samples can be obtained by open biopsies during surgical procedures. This has the benefits of enabling visualisation of the muscle extract prior to excision and allows for an increase in extract size and/or more controlled sample size in comparison to needle biopsy techniques (Derry et al., 2009; Edwards et al., 1983). In these instances patients are usually under general anaesthetic and a muscle sample is taken from a pre-existing surgical incision, removing the need for an additional surgical incision and superficial trauma. Despite this, it is typically accepted that the needle biopsy procedure presents a more efficient means of obtaining a muscle biopsy (Derry et al., 2009; Edwards et al., 1983).

In our hands, skeletal muscle extracts are obtained from patients undergoing routine bariatric surgery for obesity or obesity and type 2 diabetes mellitus by the attending surgeon. In brief, patients undergo a 12-18 hour fast prior to surgery. They are anaesthetised via short acting propofol and maintained via a volatile anaesthetic mixture of fentanyl and rocuronium. Skeletal muscle extracts are obtained via surgical excision from the *rectus abdominis* muscle by the attending surgeon (McAinch et al., 2007). Skeletal muscle samples extracted from donors to be used for cell culture are trimmed of any visible fat or connective tissue and approximately 50 mg of the muscle biopsy is suspended in serum-free alpha minimum essential media (Gibco, distributed by Invitrogen, Carlsbad, CA). These samples are immediately placed on ice for transportation and undergo no further processing prior to satellite cell isolation. Muscle samples stored in cell culture medium can be maintained at 4 °C for up to 24 hours prior to isolation of the satellite cell population with minimal adverse effects on cellular yield and viability (Blau & Webster, 1981).

4. Tissue culture methods

4.1 Isolation of myogenic satellite cells

The myogenic satellite cell population of skeletal muscle fibres was first characterised by Mauro in 1961. This study correctly identified and proposed satellite cells to be important in muscle regeneration and growth (Mauro, 1961). Degenerative myopathies or muscle injury stimulates quiescent satellite cells to re-enter the cell cycle (Charge & Rudnicki, 2004). Active satellite cells proliferate rapidly promoting muscle regeneration. Therefore controlled growth of satellite cells is seen to be favourable in the treatment of myopathies and in tissue engineering processes.

Here we describe the process of isolation of these myogenic satellite cells from skeletal muscle extracts which is modified from the methods of Blau & Webster (1981). These methods have been adapted by our laboratory in accordance with optimisation by Gaster et al., (2001a). All processing of skeletal muscle extracts for cell culture should be carried out in a sterile isolated environment, free of biological contaminants. Accordingly, biological safety cabinets should be sterilised under UV light for 20 minutes and cleaned with 70% ethanol prior to use to minimise the risk of contaminating the sample with extraneous cell types. All equipment used must be sterilised.

Satellite cells are isolated from skeletal muscle extracts of 50-100 mg through enzymatic dissociated in 0.05% trypsin-EDTA (Gibco, distributed by Invitrogen, Carlsbad, CA) via a series of incubations. Skeletal muscle extracts are washed twice in approximately 5 ml of alpha minimum essential medium and then washed 3 times in approximately 5 ml of ice-cold 1x Dulbecco's phosphate buffered saline (Gibco, distributed by Invitrogen, Carlsbad, CA). Any remaining connective tissue is removed at this stage. Subsequently, the skeletal muscle extract is manually homogenised in 3 ml of 0.05% trypsin-EDTA in a tissue culture dish using a sterile scalpel. The desired size for muscle fragments is less than 1 mm^3 (Blau & Webster, 1981). The resultant homogenate is then combined with an additional 12 ml of 0.05% trypsin-EDTA in a sterile vial, sealed and agitated on an orbital mixer for 20 minutes. Thereafter, the supernatant is aspirated and combined with 5 ml of foetal bovine serum in a 50 ml falcon tube before being placed on ice. Care must be taken at this step to ensure the finely homogenised muscle extract is not aspirated with the supernatant. An additional 15 ml of 0.05% trypsin-EDTA is added to the extract and again agitated as specified above for 20 minutes. The supernatant is combined with the initial yield in the 5 ml of foetal bovine serum. Three repetitions of this process are necessary to fully dissociate the muscle fibres. The supernatant (trypsin and foetal bovine serum mixture) is next filtered through a BD Falcon™ 100-µm nylon cell strainer (BD Biosciences, Bedford, MA). To isolate the cellular fraction of the supernatant, it is transferred to a sterile 50 ml falcon tube and is centrifuged for 7 minutes at 0.5 x g. The resulting pellet of cells will localise at the bottom of the tube and appear reddish-brown in colour. The cellular fraction is gently resuspended in 5 ml of growth medium (alpha minimum essential medium supplemented with 10% foetal bovine serum (v/v), 0.5% penicillin streptomycin (v/v) (Gibco, distributed by Invitrogen, Carlsbad, CA) and 0.5% amphotericin B (v/v) (Sigma-Aldrich, St Louis, MO)) via repeated pipette mixing.

Following the above protocol should yield approximately 5×10^3 viable, proliferating satellite cells from a 0.1 cm^3 muscle sample (Blau & Webster, 1981).

4.2 Myoblast culture and maintenance

As the cellular population isolated does not consist solely of myogenic satellite cells, the cell suspension is initially cultured on an uncoated 25 cm^2 tissue culture flask (Greiner Bio-One, Monroe, NC) for 20 minutes in a controlled humidified environment of 37 °C and 5% carbon dioxide. This increases the satellite cell content of the cultured sample and minimises contamination by fibroblasts which preferentially adhere to the surface of the tissue culture vessel. Gaster et al., (2001a) provide evidence of increased sample purity after pre-plating showing a time dependent increase in satellite cell fraction. However, increased duration of pre-plating is associated with a greater total loss of satellite cells and therefore we choose a duration of 20 minutes. After the 20 minute incubation period, gently aspirate the cell suspension taking care not to disturb the base of the flask to which the majority of fibroblasts will have attached. This flask is then discarded. The aspirated cell suspension is then seeded onto a 25 cm^2 flask coated with an extracellular matrix (Geltrex™ Reduced Growth Factor Basement Membrane Matrix; Invitrogen, Carlsbad, CA; allow extracellular matrix coating to dry in a sterile environment before seeding cells) to simulate the basement membrane under endogenous conditions. Extracellular matrices containing laminin and collagen IV, such as Geltrex™, have been shown to promote preferential satellite cells adhesion over fibroblast adhesion to enhance the satellite cell fractional content (Kuhl et al., 1986). Cells are then incubated in a cell culture CO_2 incubator in the conditions described above. Viable cells will adhere to the coated base of the tissue culture flask over the next 24 hours. These cells are considered to be at passage 1. The isolation and initial culturing of the myogenic satellite cells is depicted in figure 1.

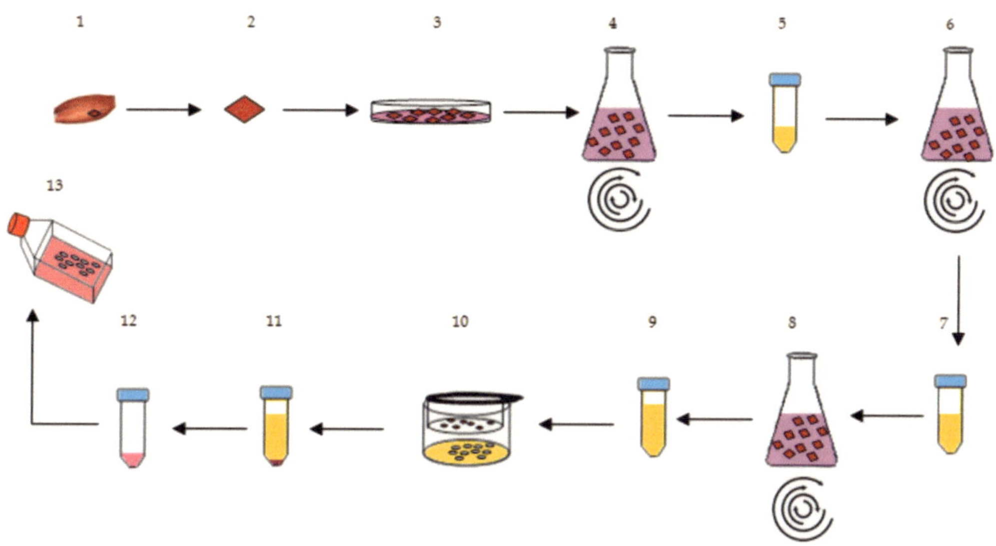

Fig. 1. Schematic representation of the isolation and initial culturing of myogenic satellite cells. 1, site of muscle biopsy is chosen; 2, biopsy extracted; 3, muscle biopsy is manually minced in trypsin-EDTA; 4, first enzymatic dissociated in trypsin under constant agitation; 5, supernatant is combined with foetal bovine serum; 6, second enzymatic dissociated in trypsin under constant agitation; 7, supernatant is combined with foetal bovine serum; 8, third enzymatic dissociated in trypsin under constant agitation; 9, supernatant is combined with foetal bovine serum; 10, supernatant/foetal bovine serum solution is filtered; 11, cellular fraction is pelleted via centrifugation, 12, cellular pellet is resuspended in growth medium; 13, isolated cells are seeded into a 25 cm^2 tissue culture flask for pre-plating and then transferred to an extracellular matrix coated flask and maintained at 37 °C and 5% carbon dioxide.

24 hours after the initial seeding, the cells are washed twice with 1x phosphate buffered saline to remove cellular debris along with non-adherent and non-viable cells. Thereafter,

growth medium (5 ml) should be refreshed every other day subsequent to a washing step with approximately 5 ml 1x phosphate buffer saline. Continue to maintain the growth of the cells until approximately 70% confluence is reached. This may take 2-3 weeks and therefore it is essential to monitor cell growth to ensure they do not become over-confluent within this period. If myoblastic cells become over-confluent, spontaneous differentiation to mature myotubes will occur and the mitogenic properties of the cells will be lost. At 70% confluency, dissociate the cells from the flask through the addition of 1.5 ml of 0.05% trypsin-EDTA and subsequent incubation at 37 °C, 5% CO_2 for 3 minutes. At this point cells will appear suspended in the media and therefore successful dissociation can be confirmed via microscopic examination. Next, inactivate the trypsin with 3 ml of growth medium, gently ejected over the base of the flask to remove any remaining adherent cells. Isolate the cellular fraction through centrifugation (5 minutes at 0.4 x g) and resuspend the cell pellet in 50 ml growth medium. Gently mix to ensure homogenous cell distribution and then seed onto five extracellular matrix coated 75 cm^2 cell culture flasks. These cells are designated to be at passage 2. Cells are again grown to approximately 70% confluent following the same procedure as describe for cells at passage 1, before dissociation and isolation via centrifugation. At this point we usually cryopreserve four of the 75 cm^2 flasks and maintain one for continued growth to passage 3. Cryopreservation enables establishment of a number of stored cell vials for future experimental use to assist in the investigation of your chosen research field. The process of cryopreservation is given in section 4.2.1. The remaining flask is passaged once more as above and seeded onto ten extracellular matrix coated 75 cm^2 flasks (split ratio 1:10). At 70% confluence cells are trypsinised and isolated via centrifugation (5 minutes at 0.4 x g) and can at this point be cryopreserved.

It is common throughout this process for cell lines isolated from different individuals to exhibit a distinct growth pattern which may be reflected in considerably longer or shorter times taken to reach confluence. Moreover, myoblasts may initially exhibit slow growth patterns, however once maintained in culture for a number of days, growth rates may increase rapidly. Therefore, regularly observing the confluence of the myoblasts is critical to ensure that passaging takes place at the appropriate confluence. Similarly to the dissociable growth patterns of myotubes derived from different individuals, myotubes may also differ in appearance depending on the donor. This can complicate the determination of confluence and therefore each cell line needs to be judged on an individual basis relative to area for growth.

4.2.1 Cryopreservation of myoblastic cells

Cryopreservation of cell stocks is an important practice in any laboratory as it helps to protect against loss of cell lines through bacterial or fungal contamination. Furthermore, as primary cell lines can be passaged finitely before becoming senescent, cryopreservation of cell lines ensures that cell stocks are maintained. It is important that viable cells are chosen for cryopreservation and that the cells are not depleted of myogenic properties due to becoming over-confluent at an earlier passage.

The cryopreservation method used in our laboratory for human primary myoblasts are described herein. Using this method we have established stocks of a large number of viable cell lines derived from muscle extracts. One 75 cm^2 flask at 70% confluent provides sufficient cells for distribution to two cryotubes. Thus, the four flasks from passage 2 can be frozen-down in eight cryotubes whilst the ten flasks from cells at passage 3 enable twenty cryotubes to be frozen. This facilitates the rapid expansion of stores of subcultures. In order to ensure consistency between studies, we cryopreserve all cells prior to experimental use. Cells are cryopreserved in a solution containing 25% growth medium (v/v), 25% foetal bovine serum (v/v) and 50% filter sterilised freezing medium. Freezing medium can be made through the addition of 10% dimethyl sulfoxide (v/v; Sigma-Aldrich, St Louis MO) to standard growth medium (as defined in section 4.1). Dimethyl sulfoxide is a freezing agent which acts to reduce the freezing point of the medium to facilitate gradual cryopreservation and prevents ice crystals forming during freezing and lysing the cells. Dimethyl sulfoxide is photosensitive and therefore it is important to protect the freezing medium from light at all stages. Freezing medium is then filter sterilised prior to use though a 0.2-μm nylon cell filter. Dissociated cells and isolate the cellular fraction via centrifugation as outlined in section 4.2 and then resuspend the pellet in growth medium (25% of total volume). Add to this the foetal bovine serum (25% of total volume). Add the pre-made freezing medium to the cell solution (50% of total volume) and gently mix. Aliquot 1 ml of this solution into each labelled cryotube. The specific volumes to be used depends on the number of flasks to be cryopreserved, however as a guide for two 75 cm^2 flask use 1 ml of growth medium, 1 ml of foetal bovine serum and 2 ml of freezing medium. To minimise cell death, cells are incrementally frozen at -20 °C for 30 minutes and then enclosed in a foam box for freezing at -80 °C overnight, before finally being stored in liquid nitrogen until required. Alternatively use a cryopreservation freezing container such as "Mr. Frosty" (Nalgene® Labware as part of Thermo Fisher Scientific, New York) which results in a controlled decrease in temperature of 1 °C per minute. Gradually decreasing the temperature during the freezing process aids in preserving cell viability and hence is critical to successful cryopreservation of a viable myoblastic cell population. However, it is also important to note that dimethyl sulfoxide is cytotoxic and therefore once cells are combined with the freezing medium it is important to progress to the freezing stage as rapidly as possible.

Conversely, the thawing procedure must take place as rapidly as possible again due to the toxic nature of dimethyl sulfoxide. We recommend immersing the bottom two thirds of the cryotube in a waterbath heated to 37 °C. Take care not to let the water reach the level of the lid as this will increase the risk of contamination of the subculture. When partially thawed the sample should be removed from the waterbath and rapidly combined with approximately 1–2 ml of growth medium to dilute the dimethyl sulfoxide and gently pipette mixed to facilitate thawing. Once fully thawed, combine the cell solution with 9 ml of growth medium and centrifuge at 0.4 x g for 5 minutes to pellet the cellular fraction. Pour off the growth medium to remove the dimethyl sulfoxide and gently resuspend the pellet in growth medium. Myoblasts can then be seeded onto 75 cm^2 or 175 cm^2 tissue culture flasks, depending on the volume of cells required for experimentation. As a rough guide one 75 cm^2 tissue culture flask at 80% confluence provides adequate cells for ten 6-well tissue culture plates or ten 100 mm tissue culture dishes. We recommend that experimentation be conducted at passage 4 or 5 to avoid senescence. For our purposes cells cryopreserved at passage 3 will be at passage 4 when thawed and subcultured. Thus at 80% confluence these cells must be seeded onto the appropriate vessel for differentiation and experimentation at passage 5. Therefore, when thawing cells it is important to be aware of the volume of cells that will be required to complete the study.

4.3 Myotube formation

The process of myoblast fusion is critical to the development of mature multinucleate skeletal muscle myotubes. During the process of myoblast differentiation, the myogenic cells exit the cell cycle and mitotic activity ceases (Linkhart et al., 1981; Yaffe, 1968). Myogenic commitment is under the synergistic regulation of a vast number of myogenic promoters (including MyoD, myogenin, Myf5, myogenic regulatory factor 4, myocyte specific enhancement factor 2) and inhibitors (including ID, Msx1, Twist and BMP-4) (reviewed by Brand-Saberi & Christ, 1999; Charge & Rudnicki, 2004). Table 1 further highlights the expression patterns of myogenic markers associated with different stages of myogenic development.

Extracellular factors also mediate myotube differentiation. Such factors include the cell-cell interactions and proximity and cellular interactions with the extracellular matrix. Concordant with this, studies by Osses & Brandan (2002) and Langen et al. (2003) show that the extracellular matrix enhances myogenic differentiation of clonal C_2C_{12} myoblasts. *In vitro*, protocols used to induce myoblast fusion vary greatly between studies. This has the potential to confound the comparison of results between studies. Predominately, differentiation protocols vary in the duration and the composition of media used to induce myogenic differentiation.

Myogenic stage	Increase expression	Decreased expression	Variable expression
Muscle derived stem cell	Sca-1 Bcl-2 All MRFs		CD34
Quiescent Satellite cell	c-MET Truncated CD34 Pax7 VCAM-1		m-cadherin Myf5 MyoD Desmin
Myogenic precursor cell	m-cadherin c-Met Full length CD34 Myf5 MyoD Desmin		Myogenin
Terminal differentiation	Myogenin MRF4 Other MRFs	CD34 Pax7	

Adapted from review by Deasy et al., (2001)
MRF; Myogenic regulatory factor.

Table 1. Expression of myogenic markers at different stages of myotube formation.

Myoblast fusion and subsequent myotube formation has been reported to occur over a period of 4-8 days (Gaster et al., 2001b). In our hands, a differentiation protocol of 4 days is sufficient to induce myoblasts elongation and fusion to produce multinucleate myotubes. The results of Gaster et al., (2001b) substantiate this, showing that on the day after culture conditions were changed to induce differentiation, myoblast fusion to form myotubes had begun and there was an increase in creatine kinase activity and fast myosin heavy chain content up until day 4 when these markers began to decline. This study also reported the presence of developing myofibrils and cross-striations at day 8 of differentiation (Gaster et al., 2001b), however no data is reported evaluating these parameters before this time. Therefore, it is hard to compare the presence of the developing contractile apparatus with functional measures such as creatine kinase activity and fast myosin heavy chain content which were seen to decline from day 4 onwards. Contrary to this Stern-Straeter et al., (2008) observed increased expression of myogenic genes from day 4 of differentiation but peaked at day 16. Creatine kinase activity in this study was also seen to peak at day 16 (Stern-Straeter et al., 2008). These results suggest a longer differentiation period may facilitate further maturation of the myotube cultures and therefore provide a more physiological representation of skeletal muscle. However, longer durations of differentiation can lead to myotube detachment and subsequent cellular death. Moreover, it has been shown in rats that the source of skeletal muscle biopsy (that is, soleus compared to extensor digitorum longus) affected the rate at which the isolated cells differentiated (Lagord et al., 1998). This suggests that the source of muscle will alter the myogenic properties of the derived human primary myotubes.

Aside from variations in the duration of culturing, myoblast fusion can be induced under a number of conditions such as a reduction in sera concentration and substitution of foetal bovine serum with horse serum, which contains less growth factors (Gaster et al., 2001a; Gaster et al., 2001b; Linkhart et al., 1981; McAinch et al., 2007). Further, addition of growth factors (vitronectin, B27 supplement, basic fibroblast growth factor, cardiotropin-1, brain-derived neitrophic factor, glial derived neurotrophic factor and neutrophin 3 and 4) (Das et al., 2009) and provision of soluble basement membrane in the absence of additional growth factors and serum (Langen et al., 2003) can also be used to promote differentiation.

In view of these variations, some contention exists as to the optimal protocol for myoblast differentiation. Accordingly, the differentiation process may need to be optimised by the end user for their specific needs. Differentiation can be confirmed via a number of different measures including analysis of sarcomere formation, creatine kinase activity, myosin heavy chain and alpha actin content and expression of myogenic markers MYoD (up-regulated in earlier stages of differentiation), myogenin, desmin, and myogenic regulatory factor 4 (Blau & Webster, 1981; Stern-Straeter et al., 2008; Stern-Straeter et al., 2007). Such analyses enable individual optimisation of the differentiation process to suit the demands of specific studies.

For our purposes the optimised differentiation protocol is as follows. At approximately 70-80% confluent, cells which have previously been seeded onto extracellular matrix coated tissue culture vessels are washed in 1x phosphate buffered saline. A simple substitution of 10% foetal bovine serum for 2% horse serum is made in the replacement medium. All other components remain the same as for the growth medium (that is, differentiation media contains 2% horse serum (v/v), 0.5% penicillin streptomycin (v/v) and 0.5% amphotericin B (v/v)). Cells are washed and differentiation media is changed every other day until day 4 is reached. When visualised microscopically cells will appear elongated and fusion will be evident. At this point myotubes are ready for experimentation.

5. Experimentation

At the conclusion of the optimised differentiation protocol, myotubes are ready for experimental purposes. However, the specific protocol used in the final stages of myotube culturing is dependent on the end use of the myotubes. That is, the way the myotubes are subcultured and subsequently lysed will depend on the experiment to be conducted. Here we will briefly examine some of the key considerations in designing experiments for analysis of different metabolic parameters.

5.1 mRNA analysis of genetic markers

The analysis of gene expression provides an invaluable source of information regarding changes in the expression of key regulatory genes. Gene expression often provides the basis for additional studies aimed at assessing the effects of experimental interventions on cellular signalling. The growth of human primary myotubes for gene expression purposes has several subtle differences to that of other outcomes. Myotubes grown for the analysis of messenger RNA abundance are typically grown in 6-well tissue culture plates (Greiner Bio-One, Monroe, NC) as decreased cell volume is typically needed for successful RNA extraction. Given the lower area for growth (approximately 9.6 cm^2 per well) confluence is often reached in a shorter period and therefore it is important to regularly check confluence to ensure differentiation is conducted at 70-80% confluence. Being over-confluent will risk the cells detaching during the experimental period. Subsequent to experimentation, the next key consideration is the process by which the cells are to be lysed. The experimental treatments should be ceased by rapidly washing each well 3 times in approximately 2 ml of ice-cold 1x phosphate buffered saline. Myotubes should be placed immediately on ice to inhibit RNase activity after the third wash and then rapidly lysed. We find the lysis of cells with TRIzol® reagent (Invitrogen, Carlsbad, CA) is highly efficient and provide a high yield of quality RNA (as determined spectrophometrically). RNA is a particularly unstable molecule and it is important to ensure that the sample is not contaminated with RNases during the extraction procedure. TRIzol® reagent acts to solubilise cellular membranes and debris whilst inhibiting RNase activity and maintains RNA integrity (Santella, 2006). However, due to the corrosive TRIzol® (including the vapour phases) cells should be transferred on ice to an RNA designated fumehood prior to the addition of this reagent. Using filtered pipette tips add 800 µl of TRIzol® to each well. Gentle agitate the TRIzol® to ensure that the entire surface of the well is covered and then repeatedly eject the TRIzol® over the base of the well to ensure myotubes are lysed. Transfer cellular lysates to a labelled tube. At this point the cellular lysates can be stored at -80 °C until ready to continue with the RNA extraction.

Total cellular RNA is then extracted through the addition of 200 µl of chloroform (Sigma Aldrich, St Louis, MO) to the cellular lysates. Mix via short vortex and then allow to sit on ice for 5 minutes. Centrifuge the TRIzol®/chloroform for 15 minutes at 16,000 x g to separate the phases. Three distinct phases should be visible; a bottom phase containing the TRIzol® and cellular debris, a thin opaque interphase and a clear RNA containing supernatant. If the separation of phases does not occur, re-vortex the tube and allow to sit on ice before centrifuging again as above. The RNA containing supernatant is then aspirated into a fresh tube containing an equal volume of isopropanol to supernatant (approximately

600 µl; Sigma Aldrich, St Louis, MO) and 10 µl of 5 M sodium chloride (Ajax Finechem, Seven Hills, Australia). Care must be taken not to contaminate the RNA sample with the interphase and therefore it is recommended that 80% of the supernatant volume be aspirated. At this point incubate the samples at -20 °C for a minimum of 2 hours (can be left overnight) to precipitate the RNA pellet. Subsequent to the incubation period, centrifuge the samples at 16,000 x g for 20 minutes to isolate the pellet. Take care to orient all tubes in the same manner to enhance the ease of RNA extraction, as the RNA pellet may be small and difficult to visualise. Aspirate the isopropanol/sodium chloride solution taking care not to aspirate the RNA pellet. Wash the pellet once with 400 µl of 75% molecular grade ethanol (Sigma Aldrich, St Louis, MO) and centrifuge for 8 minutes at 8,000 x g. Again aspirate the ethanol taking care not to aspirate the RNA pellet and then allow the pellet to air-dry for 5-8 minutes on ice. Resuspend the RNA pellet in 5 µl of sterile diethylpyrocarbonate treated water (Invitrogen, Carlsbad, CA). The resuspension of the pellet can be enhanced by heating the diethylpryocarbonate treated water to 65 °C. Transfer 1 µl of RNA to a fresh tube containing 19 µl of diethylpyrocarbonate treated water for spectrophotometric determination of RNA content at 260 nm and 280 nm. RNA purity can be determined from OD260/OD280 ratio. Samples with an OD260:OD280 ratio of 1.9 - 2.1 can be considered of high quality and relatively free of contaminates (Santella, 2006). RNA samples should be stored at -80 °C until required.

RNA can then be reverse transcribed to complementary DNA via the use of such kits as the iScript cDNA synthesis kit (Bio-Rad Laboratories, Hercules, CA). Resultant complementary DNA can then analysed for messenger RNA expression of genes of interest by such techniques as 'real-time' polymerase chain reaction (Heid et al., 1996). Data from 'real-time' polymerase chain reaction can be analysed by either absolute quantification or relative quantification (Livak & Schmittgen, 2001). Absolute quantification determines the input copy number of the gene of interest usually against known standards, whilst relative quantification enables determination of the expression of the gene of interest relative to a reference gene (Livak & Schmittgen, 2001).

5.2 Protein

The growth of myotubes for analysis of protein markers requires a greater cell density than is required for analysis of gene expression. Accordingly, when growing for analysis of protein expression, myotubes should be subcultured and grown to confluence on 100 mm tissue culture dishes (Greiner Bio-One, Monroe, NC) coated with extracellular matrix prior to differentiation. As for messenger RNA analysis cells destined for protein expression studies need to be differentiated at approximately 70-80% confluence to ensure an adequate yield. To stop experimental treatments cells should be washed twice with ice-cold 1x phosphate buffered saline. To avoid dilution of the protein fraction it is important to remove excess phosphate buffered saline with either suction or transfer pipettes. When lysing cells for protein expression the addition of a protease inhibitor to the lysis buffer is necessary to inhibit proteolytic protein degradation. For muscle cultures we find that an immunoprecipitation lysis buffer (10 mM Tris pH 7.5, 5 mM EDTA, 150 mM NaCl, 1% NP-40) containing complete mini protease inhibitor cocktail tablet per 10 ml working stock (Roche Diagnostics, Indianapolis, IN) is suitable in lysing cells for protein extraction.

Adherent skeletal muscle myotubes are lysed using 100 µl of immunoprecipitation lysis buffer and complete mini-protease inhibitor cocktail tablet. Mechanically detached adherent cells from the base of the 100 mm cell culture dish with a cell scraper (Greiner Bio-One, Monroe, NC). To proceed with protein extraction, centrifuge the cellular lysate at 17,000 x g for 4 minutes. Carefully aspirate the supernatant, aliquot and store at -80 °C. Freeze-thaw cycles should be avoided.

Protein abundance can then be quantified against known albumin standards with a working range of 20-2000 µg/ml in accordance with the assay microplate procedure using a Pierce Bicinchoninic Acid kit (Pierce Biotechnology distributed by Thermo Fisher Scientific, Scoresby, Australia) at 562 nm. We have previously found that the protein content from a single 100 mm tissue culture dish is low and in order to have sufficient protein to measure multiple markers it may be necessary to have a number of replicates for each experimental condition which can be combined to increase the overall protein concentration. If this is the case up to four 100 mm dishes can be lysed using 100 µl of lysis buffer transferred from plate to plate along with the cellular lysates. This helps to reduce sample dilution with the lysis buffer.

5.3 Glucose and fatty acid uptake

Aberrant glucose and fatty acid metabolism is observed in human primary myotubes isolated from individuals with obesity and type 2 diabetes mellitus compared to control (Bell et al., 2010; Mott et al., 2000; Thompson et al., 1996). Therefore, determination of glucose and fatty acid uptake in these cells can be a useful tool in screening new pharmacological agents aimed at ameliorating perturbed substrate metabolism. The process described below outlines the key methodological considerations for growing human primary myotubes for glucose and fatty acid uptake assays.

5.3.1 Glucose uptake

Prior to differentiation, skeletal muscle myotubes should be grown to approximately 70% confluence in 12 well tissue culture plates. At confluence, differentiation should be undertaken for 4 days. Previous results indicate that basal glucose uptake decreases upon myoblast fusion (Klip et al., 1984; Mitsumoto et al., 1991). In contrast insulin-stimulated glucose uptake increases subsequent to myoblast fusion particularly in the serum deprived L6 myotubes (Klip et al., 1984; Mitsumoto et al., 1991). Therefore for this particular assay we recommend a differentiation period of 4 days however this may need to be optimised depending on the specific outcome of the study. The protocol for measuring glucose uptake is adapted from that of Ciaraldi et al., (1995).

At confluence, myotubes are pre-incubated in serum free alpha-minimum essential medium for 4 hours and subsequently washed three times in uptake buffer (150 mM NaCl, 5 mM KCL, 1.2 mM $MgSO_4$, 2.5 mM NaH_2PO_4, 1.2 mM $CaCl_2$, 10 mM HEPES, 0.1% bovine serum albumin, pH 7.4). Myotubes should then be incubated with the compound of interest in 1 ml of uptake buffer for the given time period. Initiate the glucose uptake reaction through the addition of radiolabelled glucose (2−[^{3}H]-deoxy-D-glucose) at 1 µCi/ml and 2-deoxy-D-glucose (Perkin Elmer, Waltham, MA) at 10 µM per well and incubate at 37 °C and 5% CO_2 for 15 minutes. Subsequently, aspirate the reaction buffer and rinse the myotubes four times rapidly with ice cold 1x phosphate buffered saline to stop the reaction. Solubilise the myotubes with 500 µl of 0.1 M sodium hydroxide for 30 minutes at room temperature. This process can be enhanced by gentle agitation. The cellular lysates should then be divided with 400 µl being combined with 4 ml of scintillation fluid in scintillation vials for determination of incorporated radiolabelled glucose. The remainder of the lysates should be used to determine cellular protein content. Non-specific glucose uptake can be determined in the presence of cytochalasin B (10 µM/l) to block glucose transporter mediated glucose uptake (Ceddia et al., 2005; Fletcher et al., 2000; Michael et al., 2001). Cytochalasin B has been shown to be a potent inhibitor of cellular glucose uptake (Kletzien et al., 1972). Non-specific glucose uptake is subtracted from the total glucose uptake values and the net glucose uptake value is expressed relative to cellular protein content in picomoles of 2-deoxy-glucose taken up by the myotubes per mg protein per minute.

5.3.2 Fatty acid uptake

The process of determining fatty acid uptake is similar to that of glucose uptake and accordingly, human primary myotubes should be grown and differentiated in the same manner. Differentiated myotubes should then be exposed to the experimental conditions. Fatty acid uptake can then be measured in the presence of [1-^{14}C] palmitate (Perkin Elmer, Waltham, MA) and non-radiolabelled palmitate (Pimenta et al., 2008). In brief, the palmitate uptake is assayed through the addition of 0.2 µCi/ml [1-^{14}C] palmitate and 20 µM non-labelled palmitate (Fediuc et al., 2008) in serum free alpha-minimum essential medium for 4 minutes. Palmitate should be conjugated to fatty acid free bovine serum albumin at a molar ratio of 1. Cells should be lysed in 500 µl of 0.1 M NaOH for 30 minutes and palmitate uptake is determined relative to cellular protein content as above.

5.4 Fatty acid oxidation

In addition to determining substrate uptake it is also possible to determine the rate of fatty acid oxidation in human primary myotubes. This allows a more thorough assessment of cellular bioenergetics as corresponding results of enhanced uptake and oxidation may be indicative of improve metabolic function, whilst results of enhanced uptake but impaired oxidation may suggest that the intervention has elicited detrimental effects. Palmitate oxidation is determined from the production of radioactive $^{14}CO_2$ from [1-^{14}C] palmitate. This outcome can be determined through measurements of radiolabelled CO_2 or water with many variations existing in technique (Fediuc et al., 2006; Fediuc et al., 2008; Pathmaperuma et al., 2010; Petersen et al., 2005; Pimenta et al., 2008; Watt et al., 2006). One such method is described herein and has been adapted from previously described work of Petersen et al., (2005) in L6 skeletal muscle myotubes.

Myotubes should be grown in 100 mm tissue culture dishes until approximately 80% confluence at which point growth medium should be substituted for differentiation medium containing 2% horse serum. On day 4 of differentiation, pre-incubate the myotubes in serum free alpha minimum essential medium contain 0.1% bovine serum albumin for 2 hours. Following a washing step with 1x phosphate buffered saline, myotubes can be exposed to experimental conditions in alpha minimum essential medium containing 0.1% foetal bovine serum (v/v), 4% fatty acid free bovine serum albumin (w/v), 0.1 mM palmitate and 2 µCi of

[1-^{14}C] palmitate with the respective experimental conditions. A 2 hour treatment period has been shown to be sufficient in determining fatty acid oxidation however the period of exposure can be modified to suit the experimental design and therefore should be optimised by the end user. Subsequent to experimental exposure 1 ml of the incubation medium is added to a 20 ml scintillation vial containing 1 ml of 1 M H_2SO_4 and a 0.5 ml microcentrifuge tube containing 1 M benzethonium hydroxide to trap liberated $^{14}CO_2$ over a one hour period. The microcentrifuge tube containing the trapped $^{14}CO_2$ is then placed in a scintillation vial and counted to determine the rate of fatty acid oxidation.

6. Future applications

6.1 Three-dimensional skeletal muscle tissue constructs

Bioengineering of skeletal muscle constructs employs the use of myogenic progenitor cells and specialised scaffolding to form three-dimensional tissue constructs. Given the limited regenerative capacity of adult skeletal muscle, bioengineered skeletal muscle provides a therapeutically relevant method of reducing morbidity associated with various myopathies. Congruent with this, the long term goal of three-dimensional tissue culturing predominately centres around the provision of viable tissue transplants for regenerative purposes after acute injury or disease for instance the fabrication of three-dimensional cardiac muscle constructs. Like adult myotubes, mature cardiac myocytes are terminally differentiated cells and thus cannot regenerate subsequent to damage. Therefore the ultimate goal of bioengineered heart muscle supports myocardial regeneration after myocardial infarction, chronic heart failure or in the repair of congenital heart defects (Eschenhagen et al., 2002). This has the potential to reduce morbidity and mortality associated with cardiovascular diseases. Surgical tissue transplants are widely used in muscle regeneration after muscle injury, however muscle transplantation is associated with significant donor site morbidity, and loss of muscle volume and function (Bach et al., 2004). Implantable bioengineered skeletal muscle constructs remove the need for large muscle extracts from healthy donor tissue and thus pre-engineered tissue constructs provide an appealing treatment method for skeletal muscle pathologies. Bian & Bursac (2008) propose distinct advantages associated with the use of bioengineered muscle constructs as being the ability to engineer constructs with architecture specific for the site of damage, the ability to precondition fabricated muscle for the specific mechanical and metabolic demands of the site and the administration of specific growth factors and hormones to support growth after implantation. However, despite these potential benefits, the field of bioengineered tissues is still in its relative infancy, with muscle constructs exhibiting morphological differences to native muscle with respect to the level of differentiation and organisation of the cell microstructure, making direct comparison with native muscle problematic (Baar, 2005).

The architectural, electrical and functional integrity of fabricated muscles must be similar to that of native muscle in order to compensate for structural and functional deficits within the endogenous muscle. Accordingly, the construct needs to be contractile, demonstrate electro-physiological stability, be flexible yet mechanically robust and have angiogenic potential. Currently, bioengineered muscle constructs are small in size with Huang et al., (2005) generating myooids of 177 ± 10.5 μm in diameter with the cross-sectional area of individual myotubes being only 10 μm. This is similar to results of Powell et al., (2002) who generated human bioartificial muscles with individual myotubes being less than 10 μM in diameter. Furthermore, the current methods of generating muscle constructs result in myooids which exhibit significant deficits in force production compared to that of native muscle (Dennis et al., 2001). The absence of fibroblasts in constructs generated from C_2C_{12} cells also resulted in a force deficit manifesting in a 35% reduction in peak twitch force after tetanic stimulation (Khodabukus & Baar, 2009). The authors noted that addition of 3T3 fibroblasts to C_2C_{12} myotubes (ratio 1:5) prior to seeding attenuated this force deficit but lead to a 50% decrease in specific force. Taken together these results imply that further work needs to be done before bioengineered muscle constructs can be used for functional regeneration of human skeletal muscle. Nonetheless, in spite of the functional limitations, much can be gained through investigations of muscle formation using three-dimensional models of myotube growth (Bach et al., 2004).

Three-dimensional skeletal muscle tissue constructs provide a useful model for the study of muscle structure and function in physiological and pathophysiological states, drug screening and gene therapy despite current limitations in their fabrication (Bach et al., 2004; Vandenburgh, 2010; Vandenburgh et al., 2008). The use of three-dimensional constructs provides a method with enhanced physiological relevance due to the relative absence of cellular monolayers within their endogenous micorenvironments. Interestingly, Larkin et al., (2006) describe a method of co-culturing pre-formed self-organising primary rat tendon constructs with isolated myoblasts in place of artificial tendons, to form a functional myotendinous junction in the three-dimensional constructs formed. Functional testing of these constructs revealed the myotendinous junction could withstand tensile forces beyond the physiological range (Larkin et al., 2006). Rivron et al., (2008) further review recent advances in the ability to generate pre-vascularised tissue constructs *in vitro* which has the capacity to readily anastamose to the host vasculature and thus can enhance viability of implanted tissue constructs. These advances within the tissue engineering field represent promising progress in the development of functional muscles for regenerative purposes.

However due to the differences between native muscle and bioengineered muscle constructs, the challenges which still exist in the formation of *de novo* skeletal muscle cannot be ignored. Specific challenges still exist in supporting growth of sufficient differentiated muscle tissue for regenerative purposes, the capacity to supply sufficient oxygen and nutrients to the core of the construct, the need for these tissue constructs to remain viable and be vascularised and innervated *in vivo* (Bach et al., 2004; Birla et al., 2005; Davis et al., 2007; Gawlitta et al., 2007). Overcoming these challenges to achieve maximal therapeutic benefits centres largely around the ability to accurately recapitulate the endogenous environment for growth *in vitro*. Strategies to enhance myoblast proliferation and differentiation to support these needs are currently in great demand. One such method may be the application of mechanical stretch during construct formation. Endogenously, the electrical impulses generated by the central nervous system are critical developmental stimuli prompting the formation of mature muscle fibres with de-innervated muscle showing reduced numbers of secondary myotubes (Ross et al., 1987). In cell culture models electrical stimulation has been shown to enhance activation of quiescent satellite cells, myoblast alignment, protein synthesis, proliferation and differentiation (Donnelly et al., 2010; Tatsumi et al., 2001; Vandenburgh & Karlisch, 1989). Sarcomere formation and the development of contractile apparatus have also been shown to be enhanced by electrical stimulation in C_2C_{12} myotubes grown in three-dimensional constructs (Langelaan et al., 2010; Park et al., 2008). An 8 day mechanical stretch/relaxation protocol in bioengineered human muscles also augmented the myofibre diameter and area suggesting adaptation to a phenotype more similar to that of native muscle (Powell et al., 2002). In line with enhanced myotube diameter, Huang et al., (2005) showed that treatment with the trophic factor insulin-like growth factor 1 significantly increased force production of myooids. In further research insulin-like growth factor 1 was shown to induce myotube hypertrophy which was associated with a concomitant increase in active force production (Vandenburgh et al., 2008). This further supports the notion that extracellular paracrine factors are also important in enhancing construct formation. Levenberg et al., (2005) also demonstrated that the co-culture of myoblasts with embryonic fibroblasts and endothelial cells promoted the formation of vessel-like structures within the resultant muscle constructs which has the capacity to advance vascularisation *in vivo*. These findings highlight the significant progress being made in relation to the field bioengineering muscle constructs which resemble native muscle.

6.1.1 Growth of bioengineered tissue constructs

The growth of three-dimensional tissue cultures relies on the manipulation of the *in vitro* environment to support self-organisation of myotubes into bioengineered constructs which resemble the basic structure of *in vivo* skeletal muscle. Parallel alignment of the myotubes along a uni-directional axis is important if force is to be generated by the construct. The ability of the muscle constructs to generate adequate force to restore muscle function is likely dependent on the provision of an extracellular matrix that facilitates interactions of myofibres in a manner similar to that of native muscle (Bian & Bursac, 2008). Several forms of scaffold can be used to support organisation including non-biodegradable and biodegradable scaffolds, of which biodegradable scaffolds are preferable as their controlled degradation supports the development of native extracellular matrix and allows for the formation of densely packed myotubes in new muscle tissue (Koning et al., 2009; Rossi et al., 2010). Biodegradable scaffolds which have been employed for myooid growth include polygycolic acid, alginate and hyaluronic acid hydrogels (Kamelger et al., 2004), fibrin (Huang et al., 2005), collagen (Hinds et al., 2011) and lamina gels (Dennis et al., 2001). Biomimetic extracellular scaffolds have been shown to enhance myotube fusion and markers of differentiation in two-dimensional cell culture models (Osses & Brandan, 2002). These findings can be extrapolated and applied to three-dimensional tissue culture and thus highlights the importance of the extracellular matrix used.

Moreover, the scaffold needs to be biocompatible if the tissue is to be implanted *in vivo* as this prevents the host's immune system initiating an immune response against the foreign substance (Rossi et al., 2010) which otherwise has the potential to increase the muscle damage sustained. Indeed, recent advances in both skeletal and cardiac muscle engineering have seen bioengineered constructs successfully implanted subcutaneously in rodents (Birla et al., 2005; Levenberg et al., 2005). Birla et al., (2005) initially cultured neonatal cardiac myocytes on laminin coated plates before the bioengineered cardiac constructs were implanted subcutaneously. The authors show the implants become vascularised and cell viability is maintained for at least 3 weeks *in vivo* (Birla et al., 2005). Levenberg et al., (2005) report similar findings with the bioengineered muscle continuing to differentiate *in vivo* and anastamoses of vessels fabricated *in vitro* with the host's vasculature, as evidenced by the presence of erythrocytes within the lumen of these vessels. Importantly, the explanted constructs showed spontaneous contractility and force production was augmented compared to *in vitro* cultured controls (Birla et al., 2005). Moreover, skeletal muscle grafts cultured in collagen/Matrigel™ hydrogel have been used in myocardial repair subsequent to infarct induced by coronary ligation which was associated with cellular differentiation and vascularisation 4 weeks after implantation (Giraud et al., 2008). These findings represent significant progression towards the end goal of developing implantable tissue constructs and are an important intersect between applications for skeletal and cardiac muscle regeneration.

An additional consideration regarding the appropriateness of various scaffolds culture techniques is the provision of sufficient bioactive signals to replicate the endogenous niche to regulate satellite cells quiescence and myoblast proliferation and differentiation. Reproducing a microenvironment which accurately emulates the endogenous niche of muscle cells is complicated by the distinctive combination of cellular, biochemical and biophysical systems which define the biochemical and structurally properties of the endogenous microenvironment (Cosgrove et al., 2009). Eberli et al., (2009) support the importance of adequately replicating the microenvironment showing that the addition of fibroblast growth factor, epidermal growth factor, dexamethasone and insulin to collagen coated dishes enhances the formation of differentiated human primary myotubes. However, this issue is confounded due to the extensiveness of the list of factors which regulate myogenesis and myotube formation.

The use of Matrigel™ (BD Biosciences San Jose, CA), a bioactive extracellular matrix derive from the mouse Engelbreth-Holm-Swarm tumour lineage may partially address this issue. Matrigel abundantly produces extracellular matrix factors which support cellular growth and differentiation (reviewed by Kleinman & Martin (2005)). Given these effects, Matrigel™ is an appealing substrate to support the fabrication of three-dimensional tissue constructs. Consistent with this, Hinds et al., (2011) found that the use of a hydrogel matrix consisting of Matrigel and fibrin enhanced myotube formation and density within the construct which was positively correlated with force production. Whilst no single extracellular matrix has been identified conclusively as superior, the use of fibrin gels with aprotinin, a plasminogen inhibitor and the naturally occurring cross-linking agent, genipin, have been shown to enhance force production and time-to-failure of constructs by way of controlled degradation of this matrix (Khodabukus & Baar, 2009). Moreover, fibrin gels provide a more flexible scaffold medium into which cells migrate and proliferate both on top of and within the fibrin gel to increased specific force production (Dennis et al., 2001; Huang et al., 2005). Furthermore, controlled fibrinolysis of the fibrin gel and secretion of extracellular matrix proteins by the muscle cells allows the muscle construct to develop a phenotype more representative of native muscle (Ross & Tranquillo, 2003). When considered in conjunction with the findings of Hinds et al., (2011) this suggests enhanced fibrin gels to be an appealing substrate for fabrication of bioengineered muscle and accordingly is the method we choose to report herein due to these advantages and also the relative inexpensiveness of substrates and ease at which myooids can be formed.

The methods described are based on previous research in skeletal muscle myotubes (Huang et al., 2005). Methods utilising C_2C_{12} myotubes have since been optimised to support an extended period for which the constructs can be maintained in culture (Khodabukus & Baar, 2009). The protocol reported below is based on the optimised procedure.

Myotubes are cultured on polydimethylsiloxane (SYLGARD 184 Elastomer kit; OBA, Dandenong, Australia) coated 35 mm tissue culture dishes or 6-well tissue culture plates. Prepare the polydimethylsiloxane according to the manufacturer's instructions in a ratio of 10:1 base to curing agent. In brief, using a syringe aspirate 1.5 ml of the base agent and slowly coat the base of each dish, taking care to avoid the formation of air bubbles. Add 150 µl of the curing agent and gently mix with the pipette tip. Allow the dish to cure for 48 hours at room temperature. This process can be quickened by incubating in a humidity-free incubator at 60 °C. Place two 6 mm long braided silk sutures (Fine Science, North Vancouver, Canada) at either end of the dish with an interposing gap of 12 mm between the end of each suture. Secure the sutures in place with 0.1 mm-diameter stainless steel minutien pins (Fine Sciences, North Vancouver, Canada) as shown in Figure 2. Place multiple pins along the length of the suture to ensure that they are firmly fixed in place.

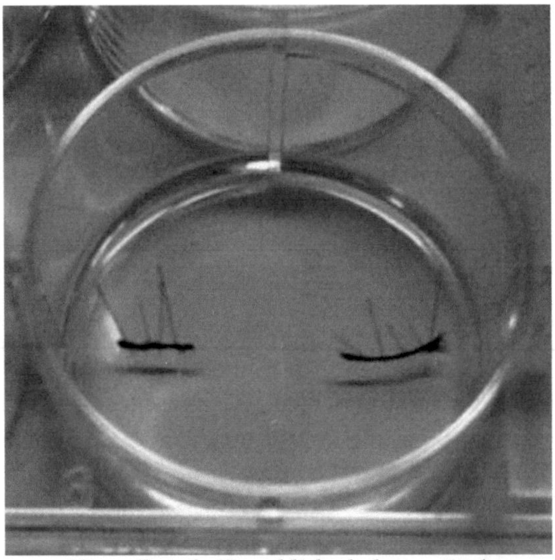

(Cornall et al., Unpublished observation)

Fig. 2. Arrangement of sutures in the polydimethylsiloxane coated well of a 6-well tissue culture plate. As the sutures are to provide the only point of force to which the myotubes align against the suture needs to be firmly affixed with multiple minutien pins along the length of the suture.

At this point it is important to sterilise the dishes to avoid contamination of the myooids constructs. This can be done by soaking the dishes in 70% ethanol for 20 minutes. Following this, aspirate the ethanol and rinse the dish with 1 ml of 1x phosphate buffered saline. The dishes can also be exposed to UV light for 1 hour to assist with sterilisation.

The next step is the preparation of the fibrin gel. Once all components have been diluted to the appropriate concentrations, determine the number of dishes and prepare a master mix of growth medium, genipin (Sigma Aldrich, St Louis, MO), thrombin (Sigma Aldrich, St Louis, MO) and aprotinin (Sigma Aldrich, St Louis, MO). C_2C_{12} myotubes growth medium is made with a base of Dulbecco's modified eagle medium supplemented with with 10% foetal bovine serum (v/v), 1% penicillin streptomyocin (v/v) and 0.5% amphotericin B. For each dish add 463 µl of growth medium containing 10 µl Genipin (stock concentration 10 mg/ml), 25 µl Thrombin (stock concentration 200 U/ ml) thrombin and 2 µl Aprotinin (stock concentration 10 mg/ ml). Gently agitate the dish until the entire surface is covered, ensure no air bubbles form around the sutures and pins. Quickly, add 200 µl of 20 mg/ml fibrinogen (Sigma Aldrich, St Louis, MO) to each dish and gently mix. Allow the gel to polymerise for 1 hour. Seed the cells into each of the dishes (100,000 cell per dish) in growth medium to a final volume of 2 ml. Allow the cells 24 hours to attach prior to changing the growth medium every other day. Myoblasts will migrate through the fibrin gel to proliferate both within and on top of the gel. After 2 days the gel should begin to contract and the myotube will begin to realign themselves between the points of force between the 2 sutures. This process should complete around day 7. The myotubes are then differentiated for 2 days in reduced serum differentiation medium (2% horse serum). Continue to maintain the forming myooids in growth medium containing 7% foetal bovine serum until construct formation is completed.

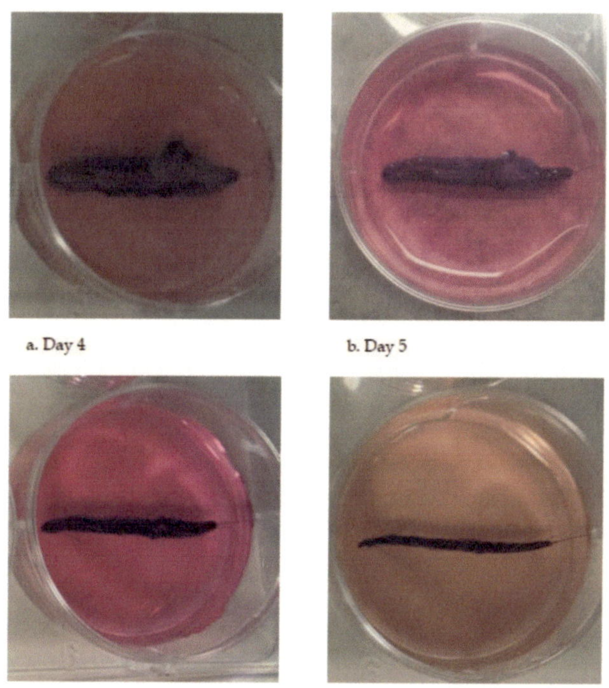

(Cornall et al., Unpublished observations)

Fig. 3. Formation of three-dimensional C_2C_{12} tissue constructs at different time points after initial seeding of the cells. Note the progressive contraction of the gel and subsequent alignment of the construct between the two sutures resulting in the formation of a densely packed three-dimensional tissue construct. At day 16 the dimensions of the construct were determined as approximately 25 mm length and 1 mm in width and the myooid was deemed to be fully formed.

Once construct formation is complete the myooids can be stimulated to contract using platinum wire electrodes positioned either side of the constructs using a force transducer. Electrical stimulation of constructs has been successfully demonstrated using clonal C_2C_{12} myotubes in a number of studies (Khodabukus & Baar, 2009; Langelaan et al., 2010; Park et al., 2008). However, in our experience the process of electrically stimulating constructs of human primary myotubes has proven difficult. Whilst we have previously been able to culture the human primary myotubes to form bioengineered skeletal muscle constructs, these myooids have been unresponsive to electrical stimulation (McAinch, Unpublished observations). As primary cells have limited myogenic capacity, this may reflect changes in the electrical potential of the membrane as the cells age in culture. It may be possible to form contractile myooids from human primary myotubes which have been isolated from the muscle sample immediately prior to culturing in this manner, as opposed to being passaged in monolayers initially. However, it remains unclear whether contractile ability is retained. Despite the lack of contractile ability, culturing the myotubes in three-dimensional arrangements provides an interesting model providing a more physiologically relevant arrangement of cells (that is, *in vivo* cells are rarely arranged in monolayers). When cultured in this manner it enables investigations into the importance of cell-cell interactions and spatial arrangements on the maturation and metabolic processes of skeletal muscle myotubes.

7. Conclusion

This chapter has highlighted the diverse nature of research applications associated with the use of human primary myotubes for studies investigating muscle physiology and the implications of this for systemic health. We have identified significant benefits of using human primary myotubes over the use of immortalised cell lines such as the C_2C_{12} and L6 cell lines due to the fact that these cells retain donor phenotypic traits. This increases the physiological relevance of results obtained in studies utilising such primary myotubes. Moreover, the relative ease at which samples of sufficient size can be obtain through simple, relatively non-invasive biopsy techniques heightens the practicality associated with their use. Whilst we have outlined the practices within our research group of isolating myogenic satellite cells, growing and maintaining myoblasts and the differentiation of myoblasts into myotubes for experimentation, it is apparent that significant variations in methodology do prevail. Therefore, the methods described in this chapter may need optimising by the end user depending on the outcomes and clinical measures of the specific study. Accordingly, we recommend these methods as a highly appropriate starting point for this procedure. We have also provided an indication of methods for a number of experimental techniques associated with the use of human primary myotubes for developing bioengineered skeletal muscle constructs and their application for the treatment of various of myopathies. This list of applications is by no means exhaustive which furthers demonstrates the versatile nature of this experimental model.

8. Acknowledgements

Lauren Cornall was supported by a scholarship (PB 10M 5472) from the National Heart Foundation of Australia. The authors would also like to acknowledge the support of the

Biomedical and Lifestyle Diseases Unit within the School of Biomedical and Health Sciences at Victoria University.

9. References

Baar, K. 2005, "New dimensions in tissue engineering: possible models for human physiology". *Exp Physiol,* 90, 799-806, 0958-0670 (Print) 0958-0670 (Linking)

Bach, A. D., Beier, J. P., Stern-Staeter, J. & Horch, R. E. 2004, "Skeletal muscle tissue engineering". *J Cell Mol Med,* 8, 413-422, 1582-1838 (Print) 1582-1838 (Linking)

Baron, A. D., Brechtel, G., Wallace, P. & Edelman, S. V. 1988, "Rates and tissue sites of non-insulin- and insulin-mediated glucose uptake in humans". *Am J Physiol,* 255, E769-774, 0002-9513 (Print) 0002-9513 (Linking)

Bell, J. A., Reed, M. A., Consitt, L. A., Martin, O. J., Haynie, K. R., Hulver, M. W., Muoio, D. M. & Dohm, G. L. 2010, "Lipid partitioning, incomplete fatty acid oxidation, and insulin signal transduction in primary human muscle cells: effects of severe obesity, fatty acid incubation, and fatty acid translocase/CD36 overexpression". *J Clin Endocrinol Metab,* 95, 3400-3410, 1945-7197 (Electronic) 0021-972X (Linking)

Berggren, J. R., Tanner, C. J. & Houmard, J. A. 2007, "Primary cell cultures in the study of human muscle metabolism". *Exerc Sport Sci Rev,* 35, 56-61, 0091-6331 (Print) 0091-6331 (Linking)

Bian, W. & Bursac, N. 2008, "Tissue engineering of functional skeletal muscle: challenges and recent advances". *IEEE Eng Med Biol Mag,* 27, 109-113, 1937-4186 (Electronic) 0739-5175 (Linking)

Birla, R. K., Borschel, G. H. & Dennis, R. G. 2005, "In vivo conditioning of tissue-engineered heart muscle improves contractile performance". *Artif Organs,* 29, 866-875, 0160-564X (Print) 0160-564X (Linking)

Blau, H. M., Pavlath, G. K., Hardeman, E. C., Chiu, C. P., Silberstein, L., Webster, S. G., Miller, S. C. & Webster, C. 1985, "Plasticity of the differentiated state". *Science,* 230, 758-766, 0036-8075 (Print) 0036-8075 (Linking)

Blau, H. M. & Webster, C. 1981, "Isolation and characterization of human muscle cells". *Proc Natl Acad Sci U S A,* 78, 5623-5627, 0027-8424 (Print) 0027-8424 (Linking)

Brand-Saberi, B. & Christ, B. 1999, "Genetic and epigenetic control of muscle development in vertebrates". *Cell Tissue Res,* 296, 199-212, 0302-766X (Print) 0302-766X (Linking)

Ceddia, R. B., Somwar, R., Maida, A., Fang, X., Bikopoulos, G. & Sweeney, G. 2005, "Globular adiponectin increases GLUT4 translocation and glucose uptake but reduces glycogen synthesis in rat skeletal muscle cells". *Diabetologia,* 48, 132-139, 0012-186X (Print) 0012-186X (Linking)

Charge, S. B. & Rudnicki, M. A. 2004, "Cellular and molecular regulation of muscle regeneration". *Physiol Rev,* 84, 209-238, 0031-9333 (Print) 0031-9333 (Linking)

Chen, M. B., Mcainch, A. J., Macaulay, S. L., Castelli, L. A., O'brien P, E., Dixon, J. B., Cameron-Smith, D., Kemp, B. E. & Steinberg, G. R. 2005, "Impaired activation of AMP-kinase and fatty acid oxidation by globular adiponectin in cultured human skeletal muscle of obese type 2 diabetics". *J Clin Endocrinol Metab,* 90, 3665-3672, 0021-972X (Print) 0021-972X (Linking)

Ciaraldi, T. P., Abrams, L., Nikoulina, S., Mudaliar, S. & Henry, R. R. 1995, "Glucose transport in cultured human skeletal muscle cells. Regulation by insulin and glucose in nondiabetic and non-insulin-dependent diabetes mellitus subjects". *J Clin Invest,* 96, 2820-2827, 0021-9738 (Print) 0021-9738 (Linking)

Condon, J., Yin, S., Mayhew, B., Word, R. A., Wright, W. E., Shay, J. W. & Rainey, W. E. 2002, "Telomerase immortalization of human myometrial cells". *Biol Reprod,* 67, 506-514, 0006-3363 (Print) 0006-3363 (Linking)

Cosgrove, B. D., Sacco, A., Gilbert, P. M. & Blau, H. M. 2009, "A home away from home: challenges and opportunities in engineering in vitro muscle satellite cell niches". *Differentiation,* 78, 185-194, 1432-0436 (Electronic) 0301-4681 (Linking)

Das, M., Rumsey, J. W., Bhargava, N., Gregory, C., Riedel, L., Kang, J. F. & Hickman, J. J. 2009, "Developing a novel serum-free cell culture model of skeletal muscle differentiation by systematically studying the role of different growth factors in myotube formation". *In Vitro Cell Dev Biol Anim,* 45, 378-387, 1543-706X (Electronic) 1071-2690 (Linking)

Davis, B. H., Schroeder, T., Yarmolenko, P. S., Guilak, F., Dewhirst, M. W. & Taylor, D. A. 2007, "An in vitro system to evaluate the effects of ischemia on survival of cells used for cell therapy". *Ann Biomed Eng,* 35, 1414-1424, 0090-6964 (Print) 0090-6964 (Linking)

Deasy, B. M., Jankowski, R. J. & Huard, J. 2001, "Muscle-derived stem cells: characterization and potential for cell-mediated therapy". *Blood Cells Mol Dis,* 27, 924-933, 1079-9796 (Print) 1079-9796 (Linking)

Dennis, R. G., Kosnik, P. E., 2nd, Gilbert, M. E. & Faulkner, J. A. 2001, "Excitability and contractility of skeletal muscle engineered from primary cultures and cell lines". *Am J Physiol Cell Physiol,* 280, C288-295, 0363-6143 (Print) 0363-6143 (Linking)

Derry, K. L., Nicolle, M. N., Keith-Rokosh, J. A. & Hammond, R. R. 2009, "Percutaneous muscle biopsies: review of 900 consecutive cases at London Health Sciences Centre". *Can J Neurol Sci,* 36, 201-206, 0317-1671 (Print) 0317-1671 (Linking)

Di Donna, S., Mamchaoui, K., Cooper, R. N., Seigneurin-Venin, S., Tremblay, J., Butler-Browne, G. S. & Mouly, V. 2003, "Telomerase can extend the proliferative capacity of human myoblasts, but does not lead to their immortalization". *Mol Cancer Res,* 1, 643-653, 1541-7786 (Print) 1541-7786 (Linking)

Dietrichson, P., Coakley, J., Smith, P. E., Griffiths, R. D., Helliwell, T. R. & Edwards, R. H. 1987, "Conchotome and needle percutaneous biopsy of skeletal muscle". *J Neurol Neurosurg Psychiatry,* 50, 1461-1467, 0022-3050 (Print) 0022-3050 (Linking)

Donnelly, K., Khodabukus, A., Philp, A., Deldicque, L., Dennis, R. G. & Baar, K. 2010, "A novel bioreactor for stimulating skeletal muscle in vitro". *Tissue Eng Part C Methods,* 16, 711-718, 1937-3392 (Electronic) 937-3384 (Linking)

Douillard-Guilloux, G., Mouly, V., Caillaud, C. & Richard, E. 2009, "Immortalization of murine muscle cells from lysosomal alpha-glucosidase deficient mice: a new tool to study pathophysiology and assess therapeutic strategies for Pompe disease". *Biochem Biophys Res Commun,* 388, 333-338, 1090-2104 (Electronic) 0006-291X (Linking)

Eberli, D., Soker, S., Atala, A. & Yoo, J. J. 2009, "Optimization of human skeletal muscle precursor cell culture and myofiber formation in vitro". *Methods,* 47, 98-103, 1095-9130 (Electronic) 1046-2023 (Linking)

Edwards, R. H., Round, J. M. & Jones, D. A. 1983, "Needle biopsy of skeletal muscle: a review of 10 years experience". *Muscle Nerve,* 6, 676-683, 0148-639X (Print) 0148-639X (Linking)

Efrat, S., Linde, S., Kofod, H., Spector, D., Delannoy, M., Grant, S., Hanahan, D. & Baekkeskov, S. 1988, "Beta-cell lines derived from transgenic mice expressing a hybrid insulin gene-oncogene". *Proc Natl Acad Sci U S A,* 85, 9037-9041, 0027-8424 (Print) 0027-8424 (Linking)

Eschenhagen, T., Didie, M., Heubach, J., Ravens, U. & Zimmermann, W. H. 2002, "Cardiac tissue engineering". *Transpl Immunol,* 9, 315-321, 0966-3274 (Print) 0966-3274 (Linking)

Fediuc, S., Gaidhu, M. P. & Ceddia, R. B. 2006, "Regulation of AMP-activated protein kinase and acetyl-CoA carboxylase phosphorylation by palmitate in skeletal muscle cells". *J Lipid Res,* 47, 412-420, 0022-2275 (Print) 0022-2275 (Linking)

Fediuc, S., Pimenta, A. S., Gaidhu, M. P. & Ceddia, R. B. 2008, "Activation of AMP-activated protein kinase, inhibition of pyruvate dehydrogenase activity, and redistribution of substrate partitioning mediate the acute insulin-sensitizing effects of troglitazone in skeletal muscle cells". *J Cell Physiol,* 215, 392-400, 1097-4652 (Electronic) 0021-9541 (Linking)

Fletcher, L. M., Welsh, G. I., Oatey, P. B. & Tavare, J. M. 2000, "Role for the microtubule cytoskeleton in GLUT4 vesicle trafficking and in the regulation of insulin-stimulated glucose uptake". *Biochem J,* 352 Pt 2, 267-276, 0264-6021 (Print) 0264-6021 (Linking)

Gaster, M., Beck-Nielsen, H. & Schroder, H. D. 2001a, "Proliferation conditions for human satellite cells. The fractional content of satellite cells". *APMIS,* 109, 726-734, 0903-4641 (Print) 0903-4641 (Linking)

Gaster, M., Kristensen, S. R., Beck-Nielsen, H. & Schroder, H. D. 2001b, "A cellular model system of differentiated human myotubes". *APMIS,* 109, 735-744, 0903-4641 (Print) 0903-4641 (Linking)

Gaster, M., Rustan, A. C., Aas, V. & Beck-Nielsen, H. 2004, "Reduced lipid oxidation in skeletal muscle from type 2 diabetic subjects may be of genetic origin: evidence from cultured myotubes". *Diabetes,* 53, 542-548, 0012-1797 (Print) 0012-1797 (Linking)

Gawlitta, D., Oomens, C. W., Bader, D. L., Baaijens, F. P. & Bouten, C. V. 2007, "Temporal differences in the influence of ischemic factors and deformation on the metabolism of engineered skeletal muscle". *J Appl Physiol,* 103, 464-473, 8750-7587 (Print) 0161-7567 (Linking)

Giraud, M. N., Ayuni, E., Cook, S., Siepe, M., Carrel, T. P. & Tevaearai, H. T. 2008, "Hydrogel-based engineered skeletal muscle grafts normalize heart function early after myocardial infarction". *Artif Organs,* 32, 692-700, 1525-1594 (Electronic) 0160-564X (Linking)

Heid, C. A., Stevens, J., Livak, K. J. & Williams, P. M. 1996, "Real time quantitative PCR". *Genome Res,* 6, 986-994, 1088-9051 (Print) 1088-9051 (Linking)

Hinds, S., Bian, W., Dennis, R. G. & Bursac, N. 2011, "The role of extracellular matrix composition in structure and function of bioengineered skeletal muscle". *Biomaterials,* 32, 3575-3583, 1878-5905 (Electronic) 0142-9612 (Linking)

Huang, Y. C., Dennis, R. G., Larkin, L. & Baar, K. 2005, "Rapid formation of functional muscle in vitro using fibrin gels". *J Appl Physiol,* 98, 706-713, 8750-7587 (Print) 0161-7567 (Linking)

Jat, P. S., Noble, M. D., Ataliotis, P., Tanaka, Y., Yannoutsos, N., Larsen, L. & Kioussis, D. 1991, "Direct derivation of conditionally immortal cell lines from an H-2Kb-tsA58 transgenic mouse". *Proc Natl Acad Sci U S A,* 88, 5096-5100, 0027-8424 (Print) 0027-8424 (Linking)

Kamelger, F. S., Marksteiner, R., Margreiter, E., Klima, G., Wechselberger, G., Hering, S. & Piza, H. 2004, "A comparative study of three different biomaterials in the engineering of skeletal muscle using a rat animal model". *Biomaterials,* 25, 1649-1655, 0142-9612 (Print) 0142-9612 (Linking)

Kessler, P. D., Podsakoff, G. M., Chen, X., Mcquiston, S. A., Colosi, P. C., Matelis, L. A., Kurtzman, G. J. & Byrne, B. J. 1996, "Gene delivery to skeletal muscle results in sustained expression and systemic delivery of a therapeutic protein". *Proc Natl Acad Sci U S A,* 93, 14082-14087, 0027-8424 (Print) 0027-8424 (Linking)

Khodabukus, A. & Baar, K. 2009, "Regulating fibrinolysis to engineer skeletal muscle from the C2C12 cell line". *Tissue Eng Part C Methods,* 15, 501-511, 1937-3392 (Electronic) 1937-3384 (Linking)

Kleinman, H. K. & Martin, G. R. 2005, "Matrigel: basement membrane matrix with biological activity". *Semin Cancer Biol,* 15, 378-386, 1044-579X (Print) 1044-579X (Linking)

Kletzien, R. F., Perdue, J. F. & Springer, A. 1972, "Cytochalasin A and B. Inhibition of sugar uptake in cultured cells". *J Biol Chem,* 247, 2964-2966, 0021-9258 (Print) 0021-9258 (Linking)

Klip, A., Li, G. & Logan, W. J. 1984, "Induction of sugar uptake response to insulin by serum depletion in fusing L6 myoblasts". *Am J Physiol,* 247, E291-296, 0002-9513 (Print) 0002-9513 (Linking)

Koning, M., Harmsen, M. C., Van Luyn, M. J. & Werker, P. M. 2009, "Current opportunities and challenges in skeletal muscle tissue engineering". *J Tissue Eng Regen Med,* 3, 407-415, 1932-7005 (Electronic) 1932-6254 (Linking)

Kuhl, U., Ocalan, M., Timpl, R. & Von Der Mark, K. 1986, "Role of laminin and fibronectin in selecting myogenic versus fibrogenic cells from skeletal muscle cells in vitro". *Dev Biol,* 117, 628-635, 0012-1606 (Print) 0012-1606 (Linking)

Lagord, C., Soulet, L., Bonavaud, S., Bassaglia, Y., Rey, C., Barlovatz-Meimon, G., Gautron, J. & Martelly, I. 1998, "Differential myogenicity of satellite cells isolated from extensor digitorum longus (EDL) and soleus rat muscles revealed in vitro". *Cell Tissue Res,* 291, 455-468, 0302-766X (Print) 0302-766X (Linking)

Langelaan, M. L., Boonen, K. J., Rosaria-Chak, K. Y., Van Der Schaft, D. W., Post, M. J. & Baaijens, F. P. 2010, "Advanced maturation by electrical stimulation: Differences in response between C2C12 and primary muscle progenitor cells". *J Tissue Eng Regen Med,* 1932-7005 (Electronic) 1932-6254 (Linking)

Langen, R. C., Schols, A. M., Kelders, M. C., Wouters, E. F. & Janssen-Heininger, Y. M. 2003, "Enhanced myogenic differentiation by extracellular matrix is regulated at the early stages of myogenesis". *In Vitro Cell Dev Biol Anim,* 39, 163-169, 1071-2690 (Print) 1071-2690 (Linking)

Larkin, L. M., Calve, S., Kostrominova, T. Y. & Arruda, E. M. 2006, "Structure and functional evaluation of tendon-skeletal muscle constructs engineered in vitro". *Tissue Eng,* 12, 3149-3158, 1076-3279 (Print) 1076-3279 (Linking)

Levenberg, S., Rouwkema, J., Macdonald, M., Garfein, E. S., Kohane, D. S., Darland, D. C., Marini, R., Van Blitterswijk, C. A., Mulligan, R. C., D'amore, P. A. & Langer, R. 2005, "Engineering vascularized skeletal muscle tissue". *Nat Biotechnol,* 23, 879-884, 1087-0156 (Print) 1087-0156 (Linking)

Linkhart, T. A., Clegg, C. H. & Hauschika, S. D. 1981, "Myogenic differentiation in permanent clonal mouse myoblast cell lines: regulation by macromolecular growth factors in the culture medium". *Dev Biol,* 86, 19-30, 0012-1606 (Print) 0012-1606 (Linking)

Livak, K. J. & Schmittgen, T. D. 2001, "Analysis of relative gene expression data using real-time quantitative PCR and the 2(-Delta Delta C(T)) Method". *Methods,* 25, 402-408, 1046-2023 (Print) 1046-2023 (Linking)

Loro, E., Rinaldi, F., Malena, A., Masiero, E., Novelli, G., Angelini, C., Romeo, V., Sandri, M., Botta, A. & Vergani, L. 2010, "Normal myogenesis and increased apoptosis in myotonic dystrophy type-1 muscle cells". *Cell Death Differ,* 17, 1315-1324, 1476-5403 (Electronic) 1350-9047 (Linking)

Machida, S., Spangenburg, E. E. & Booth, F. W. 2004, "Primary rat muscle progenitor cells have decreased proliferation and myotube formation during passages". *Cell Prolif,* 37, 267-277, 0960-7722 (Print) 0960-7722 (Linking)

Macpherson, P. C., Suhr, S. T. & Goldman, D. 2004, "Activity-dependent gene regulation in conditionally-immortalized muscle precursor cell lines". *J Cell Biochem,* 91, 821-839, 0730-2312 (Print) 0730-2312 (Linking)

Mauro, A. 1961, "Satellite cell of skeletal muscle fibers". *J Biophys Biochem Cytol,* 9, 493-495, 0095-9901 (Print) 0095-9901 (Linking)

Mcainch, A. J. & Cameron-Smith, D. 2009, "Adiponectin decreases pyruvate dehydrogenase kinase 4 gene expression in obese- and diabetic-derived myotubes". *Diabetes Obes Metab,* 11, 721-728, 1463-1326 (Electronic) 1462-8902 (Linking)

Mcainch, A. J., Steinberg, G. R., Chen, M. B., O'brien, P. E., Dixon, J. B., Cameron-Smith, D. & Kemp, B. E. 2006a, "The suppressor of cytokine signaling 3 inhibits leptin activation of AMP-kinase in cultured skeletal muscle of obese humans". *J Clin Endocrinol Metab,* 91, 3592-3597, 0021-972X (Print) 0021-972X (Linking)

Mcainch, A. J., Steinberg, G. R., Mollica, J., O'brien, P. E., Dixon, J. B., Macaulay, S. L., Kemp, B. E. & Cameron-Smith, D. 2006b, "Differential regulation of adiponectin receptor gene expression by adiponectin and leptin in myotubes derived from obese and diabetic individuals". *Obesity (Silver Spring),* 14, 1898-1904, 1930-7381 (Print)

Mcainch, A. J., Steinberg, G. R., Mollica, J., O'brien, P. E., Dixon, J. B., Kemp, B. E. & Cameron-Smith, D. 2007, "Leptin stimulation of COXIV is impaired in obese skeletal muscle myotubes". *Obes Res Clin Pract,* 1, 53-60, 1871-403X

Melendez, M. M., Vosswinkel, J. A., Shapiro, M. J., Gelato, M. C., Mynarcik, D., Gavi, S., Xu, X. & Mcnurlan, M. 2007, "Wall suction applied to needle muscle biopsy - a novel technique for increasing sample size". *J Surg Res,* 142, 301-303, 0022-4804 (Print) 0022-4804 (Linking)

Michael, L. F., Wu, Z., Cheatham, R. B., Puigserver, P., Adelmant, G., Lehman, J. J., Kelly, D. P. & Spiegelman, B. M. 2001, "Restoration of insulin-sensitive glucose transporter

(GLUT4) gene expression in muscle cells by the transcriptional coactivator PGC-1". *Proc Natl Acad Sci U S A,* 98, 3820-3825, 0027-8424 (Print) 0027-8424 (Linking)

Mitsumoto, Y., Burdett, E., Grant, A. & Klip, A. 1991, "Differential expression of the GLUT1 and GLUT4 glucose transporters during differentiation of L6 muscle cells". *Biochem Biophys Res Commun,* 175, 652-659, 0006-291X (Print) 0006-291X (Linking)

Mott, D. M., Hoyt, C., Caspari, R., Stone, K., Pratley, R. & Bogardus, C. 2000, "Palmitate oxidation rate and action on glycogen synthase in myoblasts from insulin-resistant subjects". *Am J Physiol Endocrinol Metab,* 279, E561-569, 0193-1849 (Print) 0193-1849 (Linking)

Obinata, M. 2001, "Possible applications of conditionally immortalized tissue cell lines with differentiation functions". *Biochem Biophys Res Commun,* 286, 667-672, 0006-291X (Print) 0006-291X (Linking)

Osses, N. & Brandan, E. 2002, "ECM is required for skeletal muscle differentiation independently of muscle regulatory factor expression". *Am J Physiol Cell Physiol,* 282, C383-394, 0363-6143 (Print) 0363-6143 (Linking)

Park, H., Bhalla, R., Saigal, R., Radisic, M., Watson, N., Langer, R. & Vunjak-Novakovic, G. 2008, "Effects of electrical stimulation in C2C12 muscle constructs". *J Tissue Eng Regen Med,* 2, 279-287, 1932-6254 (Print) 1932-6254 (Linking)

Pathmaperuma, A. N., Mana, P., Cheung, S. N., Kugathas, K., Josiah, A., Koina, M. E., Broomfield, A., Delghingaro-Augusto, V., Ellwood, D. A., Dahlstrom, J. E. & Nolan, C. J. 2010, "Fatty acids alter glycerolipid metabolism and induce lipid droplet formation, syncytialisation and cytokine production in human trophoblasts with minimal glucose effect or interaction". *Placenta,* 31, 230-239, 1532-3102 (Electronic) 0143-4004 (Linking)

Petersen, E. W., Carey, A. L., Sacchetti, M., Steinberg, G. R., Macaulay, S. L., Febbraio, M. A. & Pedersen, B. K. 2005, "Acute IL-6 treatment increases fatty acid turnover in elderly humans in vivo and in tissue culture in vitro". *Am J Physiol Endocrinol Metab,* 288, E155-162, 0193-1849 (Print) 0193-1849 (Linking)

Pimenta, A. S., Gaidhu, M. P., Habib, S., So, M., Fediuc, S., Mirpourian, M., Musheev, M., Curi, R. & Ceddia, R. B. 2008, "Prolonged exposure to palmitate impairs fatty acid oxidation despite activation of AMP-activated protein kinase in skeletal muscle cells". *J Cell Physiol,* 217, 478-485, 1097-4652 (Electronic) 0021-9541 (Linking)

Powell, C. A., Smiley, B. L., Mills, J. & Vandenburgh, H. H. 2002, "Mechanical stimulation improves tissue-engineered human skeletal muscle". *Am J Physiol Cell Physiol,* 283, C1557-1565, 0363-6143 (Print) 0363-6143 (Linking)

Richler, C. & Yaffe, D. 1970, "The in vitro cultivation and differentiation capacities of myogenic cell lines". *Dev Biol,* 23, 1-22, 0012-1606 (Print) 0012-1606 (Linking)

Ridley, A. J., Paterson, H. F., Noble, M. & Land, H. 1988, "Ras-mediated cell cycle arrest is altered by nuclear oncogenes to induce Schwann cell transformation". *EMBO J,* 7, 1635-1645, 0261-4189 (Print) 0261-4189 (Linking)

Rivron, N. C., Liu, J. J., Rouwkema, J., De Boer, J. & Van Blitterswijk, C. A. 2008, "Engineering vascularised tissues in vitro". *Eur Cell Mater,* 15, 27-40, 1473-2262 (Electronic) 1473-2262 (Linking)

Ross, J. J., Duxson, M. J. & Harris, A. J. 1987, "Neural determination of muscle fibre numbers in embryonic rat lumbrical muscles". *Development,* 100, 395-409, 0950-1991 (Print) 0950-1991 (Linking)

Ross, J. J. & Tranquillo, R. T. 2003, "ECM gene expression correlates with in vitro tissue growth and development in fibrin gel remodeled by neonatal smooth muscle cells". *Matrix Biol,* 22, 477-490, 0945-053X (Print) 0945-053X (Linking)

Rossi, C. A., Pozzobon, M. & De Coppi, P. 2010, "Advances in musculoskeletal tissue engineering: moving towards therapy". *Organogenesis,* 6, 167-172, 1555-8592 (Electronic) 1547-6278 (Linking)

Santella, R. M. 2006, "Approaches to DNA/RNA Extraction and whole genome amplification". *Cancer Epidemiol Biomarkers Prev,* 15, 1585-1587, 1055-9965 (Print) 1055-9965 (Linking)

Steinberg, G. R., Mcainch, A. J., Chen, M. B., O'brien, P. E., Dixon, J. B., Cameron-Smith, D. & Kemp, B. E. 2006, "The suppressor of cytokine signaling 3 inhibits leptin activation of AMP-kinase in cultured skeletal muscle of obese humans". *J Clin Endocrinol Metab,* 91, 3592-3597, 0021-972X (Print) 0021-972X (Linking)

Stern-Straeter, J., Bran, G., Riedel, F., Sauter, A., Hormann, K. & Goessler, U. R. 2008, "Characterization of human myoblast cultures for tissue engineering". *Int J Mol Med,* 21, 49-56, 1107-3756 (Print) 1107-3756 (Linking)

Stern-Straeter, J., Riedel, F., Bran, G., Hormann, K. & Goessler, U. R. 2007, "Advances in skeletal muscle tissue engineering". *In Vivo,* 21, 435-444, 0258-851X (Print) 0258-851X (Linking)

Tarnopolsky, M. A., Pearce, E., Smith, K. & Lach, B. 2011, "Suction-modified Bergstrom muscle biopsy technique: experience with 13,500 procedures". *Muscle Nerve,* 43, 717-725, 1097-4598 (Electronic) 0148-639X (Linking)

Tatsumi, R., Sheehan, S. M., Iwasaki, H., Hattori, A. & Allen, R. E. 2001, "Mechanical stretch induces activation of skeletal muscle satellite cells in vitro". *Exp Cell Res,* 267, 107-114, 0014-4827 (Print) 0014-4827 (Linking)

Thompson, D. B., Pratley, R. & Ossowski, V. 1996, "Human primary myoblast cell cultures from non-diabetic insulin resistant subjects retain defects in insulin action". *J Clin Invest,* 98, 2346-2350, 0021-9738 (Print) 0021-9738 (Linking)

Todaro, G. J. & Green, H. 1963, "Quantitative studies of the growth of mouse embryo cells in culture and their development into established lines". *J Cell Biol,* 17, 299-313, 0021-9525 (Print) 0021-9525 (Linking)

Todaro, G. J., Nilausen, K. & Green, H. 1963, "Growth Properties of Polyoma Virus-Induced Hamster Tumor Cells". *Cancer Res,* 23, 825-832, 0008-5472 (Print) 0008-5472 (Linking)

Vandenburgh, H. 2010, "High-content drug screening with engineered musculoskeletal tissues". *Tissue Eng Part B Rev,* 16, 55-64, 1937-3376 (Electronic) 1937-3368 (Linking)

Vandenburgh, H., Shansky, J., Benesch-Lee, F., Barbata, V., Reid, J., Thorrez, L., Valentini, R. & Crawford, G. 2008, "Drug-screening platform based on the contractility of tissue-engineered muscle". *Muscle Nerve,* 37, 438-447, 0148-639X (Print) 0148-639X (Linking)

Vandenburgh, H. H. & Karlisch, P. 1989, "Longitudinal growth of skeletal myotubes in vitro in a new horizontal mechanical cell stimulator". *In Vitro Cell Dev Biol,* 25, 607-616, 0883-8364 (Print) 0883-8364 (Linking)

Watt, M. J., Steinberg, G. R., Chen, Z. P., Kemp, B. E. & Febbraio, M. A. 2006, "Fatty acids stimulate AMP-activated protein kinase and enhance fatty acid oxidation in L6 myotubes". *J Physiol,* 574, 139-147, 0022-3751 (Print) 0022-3751 (Linking)

Yaffe, D. 1968, "Retention of differentiation potentialities during prolonged cultivation of myogenic cells". *Proc Natl Acad Sci U S A,* 61, 477-483, 0027-8424 (Print) 0027-8424 (Linking)

Yaffe, D. & Saxel, O. 1977, "Serial passaging and differentiation of myogenic cells isolated from dystrophic mouse muscle". *Nature,* 270, 725-727, 0028-0836 (Print) 0028-0836 (Linking)

Zurlo, F., Larson, K., Bogardus, C. & Ravussin, E. 1990, "Skeletal muscle metabolism is a major determinant of resting energy expenditure". *J Clin Invest,* 86, 1423-1427, 0021-9738 (Print) 0021-9738 (Linking)

4

Membrane Transport in Human Skeletal Muscle

Carsten Juel
University of Copenhagen
Denmark

1. Introduction

Membrane transport in human skeletal muscle can be studied with different techniques ranging from whole body exercise experiments to *in vitro* experiments with membranes obtained from human skeletal muscle. The membranes for these experiments are usually obtained with the biopsy technique.

2. Muscle biopsy

A muscle biopsy is a small sample of muscle. Theoretically this sample could be obtained by surgery. However, in muscle physiology the established method is the needle-biopsy method, usually called the Bergström technique (Bergström 1962). With this technique it is possible to obtain 10-100 mg wet weight of tissue or even more if suction is applied.

2.1 Use of muscle biopsies

In exercise physiology biopsies obtained before and after exercise have been used to obtain snapshoots of the muscle content of ions and metabolites. For instance, the changes in muscle glycogen and glucose in association with muscle activity have been quantified. Changes in ion composition, for instance accumulation of lactic acid in muscle, the associated changes in pH, and changes in Na^+ and K^+ distribution have also been of interest. By repeated biopsies it has been possible to describe the recovery processes after exercise. Such measurements are usually combined with blood analysis of the same ions or metabolites (see exercise experiments below).

Muscle biopsies have also been used to obtain snapshoots of the active genes. Measurements of transcriptional activity in human skeletal muscle have been difficult because of the large amount of muscle tissue needed to isolate nuclei. A new technique involving RT-PCR for performing nuclear "run-on" analysis made it possible to determine transcriptional activity in the small amount of tissue available from a needle biopsy. This opened the possibility to measure transcriptional activity before and in the recovery period in association with muscle activity (Pilegaard et al. 2000, Hildebrand & Neufer, 2000).

2.2 Scope of the paper

The present review focuses on the use of biopsy material in studies of membrane transport in animals and especially in humans. The use of biopsy analysis and vesicles produced from biopsies will be reviewed. It will be described that information obtained with this technique can be combined with information obtained from whole body experiments.

3. Membrane transport in general

3.1 Specific transport systems

Membrane transport involves all types of protein-mediated transport systems, including channels, carriers, exchangers and pumps.

3.1.1 Vesicle studies

In animal studies it is possible to use isolated muscle for transport studies. If a muscle is incubated with a radiolabeled compound it is possible to show uptake, and if specific inhibiters are known, it is possible to demonstrate that the uptake is mediated by specific membrane transport systems. However, a muscle consists of a high number of cells, it is therefore not possible to incubate all cells at the same time point, to control the gradient and to measure initial rate of uptake. It is therefore not possible based on intact muscle to determine the transport kinetic parameters K_m and V_{max}, the Michaelis- Menten parameters. In addition, this type of measurements can not be done in humans.

The use of vesicles made from human biopsies has solved these problems.

It has been known for long time that if tissue is homogenized, the membranes usually form small closed structures, called vesicles. The diameter of these vesicles is usually less than 0.5 µm. Such vesicles have been used for transport studies, but they are difficult to use because of the fast uptake/release of compounds due to the large surface/volume ration.

Sarcolemmal giant vesicles are produced with a different method (Burton & Hutter, 1990). Muscles are cut in pieces (but are not homogenized), the pieces are treated with collagenase and a high K^+ concentration (Juel 1991). The exact mechanism is not known. The effect of high potassium could be due to an osmotic gradient, bud this is difficult to accept because the cells are not intact. Anyway, the outer membranes but out and form large vesicles, which can be purified using a step density gradient and slow centrifugation. The purified vesicles are from 1-50 µm, with a median of 6 µm (Figure 1). This is the size of a red blood cell. Experiments with labeling of the extracellular part of the Na,K-ATPase with ouabain have shown no additional labeling if the vesicles were opened, which implies that the original outside is still facing outwards, this is usually called right side out. These vesicles are much better suited for transport studies because of the lower surface-volume ration. In the next sections this type of vesicles will be called sarcolemmal giant vesicles.

It must be noted that this type of vesicles can only be produced from fresh muscle material; vesicles can not be produced from frozen material.

Other types of vesicles have been called giant vesicles; in the present paper the name sarcolemmal giant vesicles is restricted to vesicles made with collagenase and K^+ treatment of muscle.

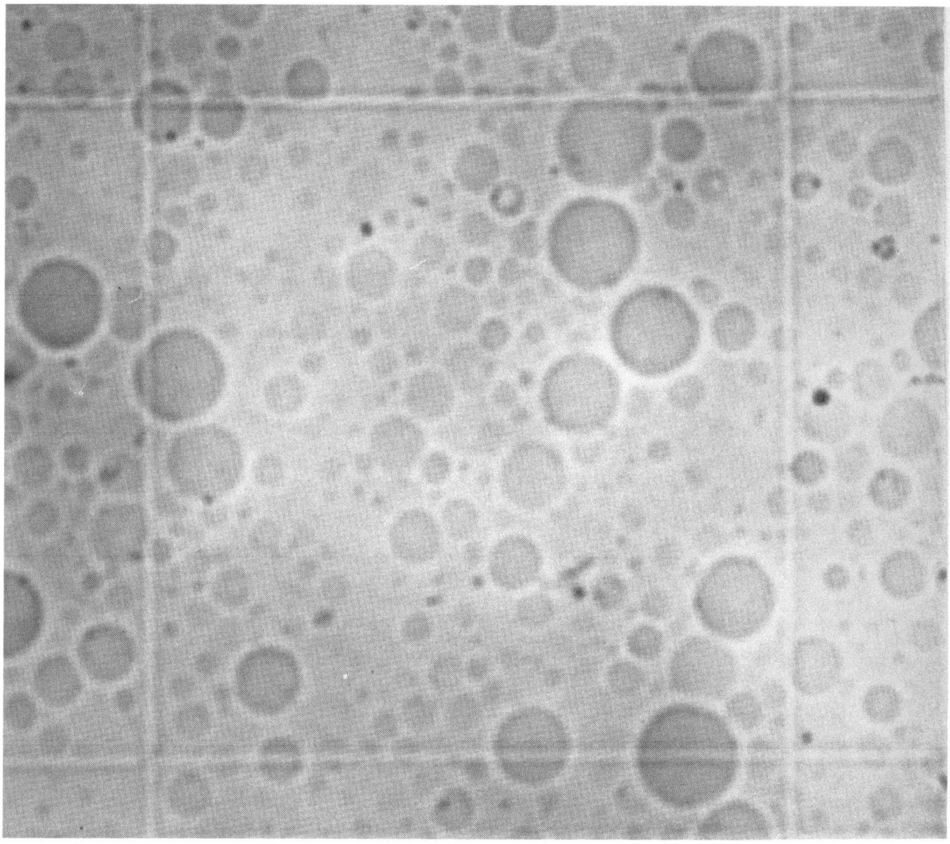

Fig. 1. Vesicles viewed in the light microscope. These vesicles were produced from human biopsy material. Grid: 200µm.

3.1.2 Lactate transport studies

Lactate transport was first described in red blood cells. Later it was shown with isolated muscle that the lactate uptake in incubated muscle can be inhibited by unspecific transport inhibitors (SH-group binding or cinnamate). But this method could not be used to obtain the Michealis-Menten parameters. The first study of lactate transport with sarcolemmal giant vesicles was carried out with vesicles produced from rat muscle. With this technique it was possible to demonstrate saturation, the effects of inhibitors, trans-acceleration, and to determine the Michaelis-Menten parameters in different experimental situation: zero-trans efflux and equilibrium exchange (Figure 2, right).

The Michaelis-Menten parameters for lactate/H^+ co-transport in human skeletal muscle were obtained with vesicles made from needle biopsies (Juel et al. 1994). This is one of the first membrane transport studies in humans. The use of vesicles made this possible. Lactate transport (quantified as tracer fluxes) was determined with different lactate concentrations in the vesicles and outside the vesicles. This setup and the use of inhibitors to quantify simple diffusion made it possible to calculate the Michaelin-Menten parameters K_m and V_{max} both for zero-trans experiments and equilibrium exchange experiments (Figure 2).

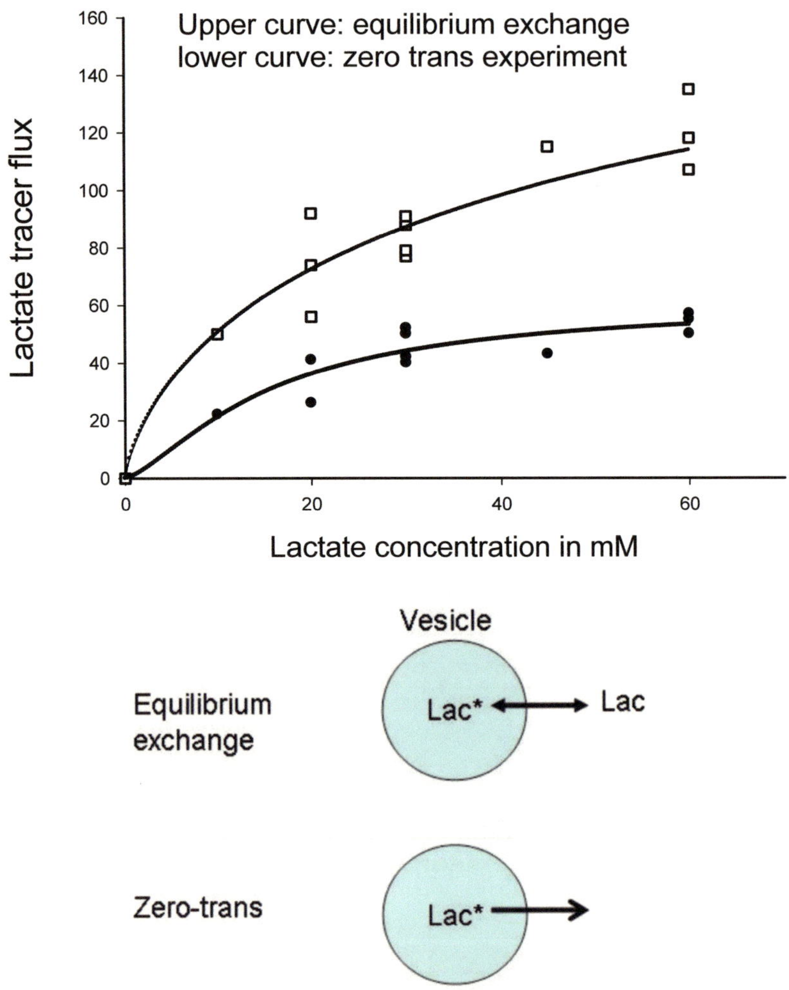

Fig. 2. Lactate transport measures in giant vesicles produced from human skeletal muscle biopsies. Data from zero-trans experiments (lactate initially present on one side of the membrane) and equilibrium exchange experiments (identical lactate concentration at both sides of the membrane, but initially with radio-labeled lactate only at one side). K_m was found to be 24 and 30 mM lactate, respectively. The lines represent Michaelis-Menten fits to the data. Adapted from Juel et al. 1994. Analysis of the pH changes in the same experiments revealed that lactate and H^+ were transported with a 1:1 ratio; lactate/H^+ co-transport is therefore the correct name for this type of transport.

3.1.3 Lactate transport and training in humans

The proteins responsible for lactate/H^+ co-transport were cloned in 1994, but antibodies for studies of the two isoforms MCT1 and MCT4 were first available in 1998 (Wilson et al. 1998). However, with the use of biopsy material and giant vesicles it was possible to investigate the effect of training before the proteins were identified. Biopsies were obtained from subjects with different training status and the rate of lactate transport was quantified from tracer fluxes across vesicular membranes (Figure 3).

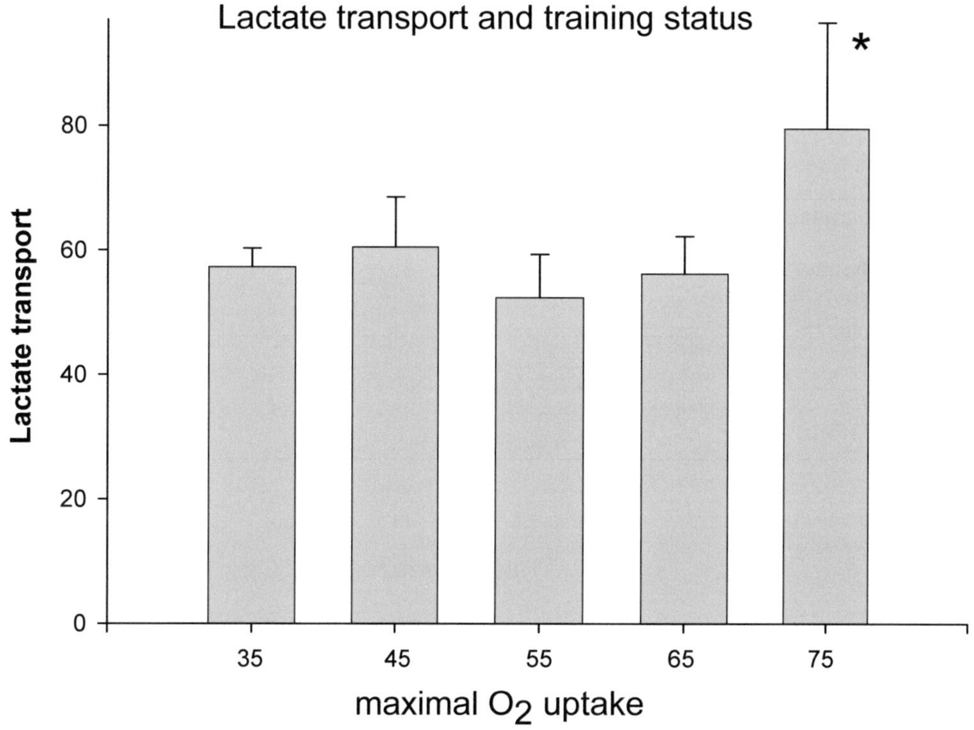

Fig. 3. Lactate transport in vesicles produced from human biopsy material. Lactate transport was quantified as tracer flux in vesicles incubated with radio-labeled lactate. Maximal O_2 uptake was used as an index of training status. It can be seen that some individuals with high training status had an improved lactate transport capacity (Data from Pilegaard et al. 1994).

It was concluded that some well trained sprinters had an increased lactate transport capacity. Later it was confirmed with antibodies and biopsy material that training can increase the protein density of the proteins involved (Pilegaard et al. 1999). Lactate/H^+ co-transport is mediated by two isoforms called MCT1 and MCT4 (for monocarboxylate transporter 1 and 4).

3.2 Exercise induced changes in transport proteins studied with muscle biopsies

3.2.1 Exercise

Muscle biopsies have also been an exceptional tool to investigate the effects of exercise training. In combination with the western blotting technique it has been possible to quantify the changes at the protein level of many transport proteins, for instance the glucose transporter, the lactate H^+ co-transporter, the Na^+/H^+ exchanger and the Na,K-pump. For a review on exercise-induced changes in muscle membrane transport systems see (Juel 2006) and Figure 4.

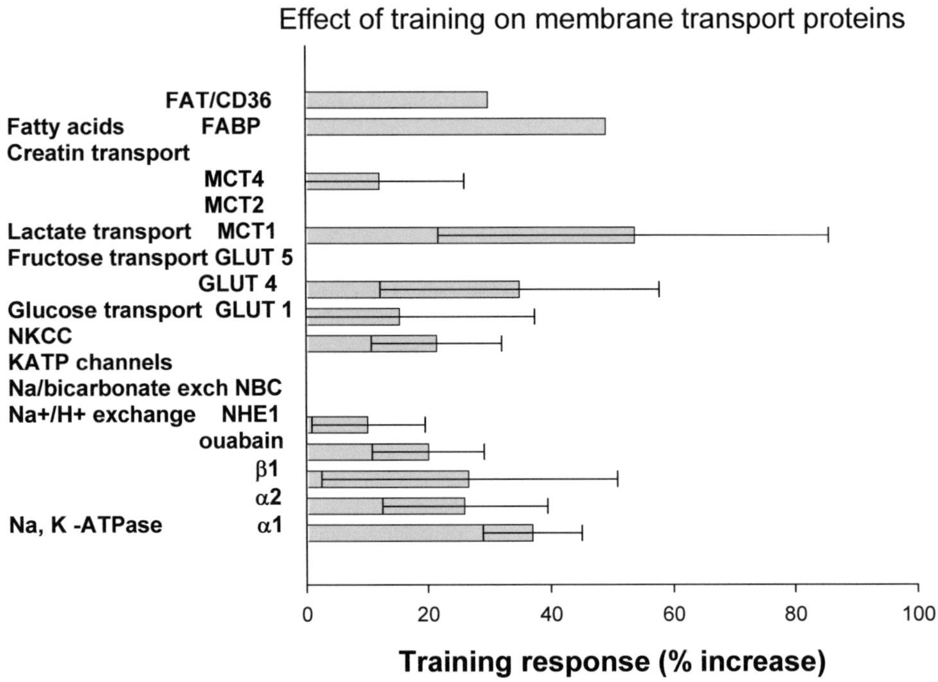

Fig. 4. Changes in membrane proteins involved in membrane transport; effect of training. All data were obtained with human muscle biopsies taken before and after a training period of various durations (weeks) and intensities. Mean ± SD if more than one study. Please note that these data are collected from training studies with different training intensities and durations. Modified from Juel 2006.

It can be concluded from Figure 4 that all membrane transport proteins studied in humans can undergo changes with training. Although this is a well known phenomenon, the exact signaling pathways from physical activity to gene transcription are only partly known.

3.2.2 Biopsies in exercise and training physiology with special focus on membrane transport in humans

The use of biopsies as snapshots of the ion and metabolite content in muscle is used in training and exercise physiology. In addition, biopsies can be used to monitor changes in proteins of importance for function. The combined used of other measurements (typically blood analysis) and biopsies in training and exercise physiology is demonstrated in the example below.

Human subjects trained with one leg for 8 weeks. The daily training consisted of fifteen 1-min high intensity bouts (150 % VO_2 max) separated by 3 min rest. After the training periods an exercise test was carried out both with the trained and the untrained leg. The test consisted of incremental exercise to exhaustion. Blood samples were obtained before, during the experiment, and in the recovery period. The releases of lactate and H^+ were calculated from the blood concentrations and blood flow. The effect of training on lactate release is illustrated in Figure 5.

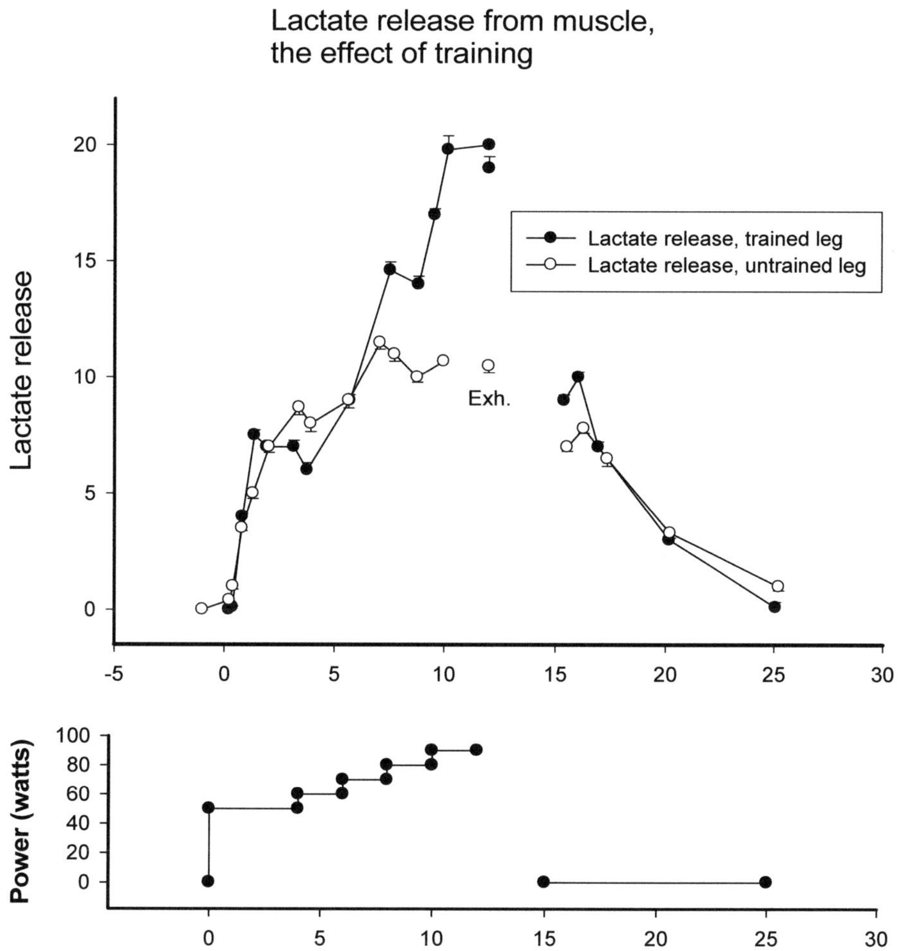

Fig. 5. Lactate release from exercising leg muscle, the effect of training. Values were calculated from arterial and venous blood lactate concentration, and blood flow. Exh: value at exhaustion. The exercise intensity (in Watts) is indicated in the diagram below. Adapted from Juel et al. 2004.

It can be concluded that lactate release was nearly doubled in the trained leg compared to the untrained leg (Juel et al. 2004). The question is now, what is the underlying mechanism? Changes in lactate release could be due to changes in the amount of lactate accumulated in the active muscle. Biopsy samples were therefore analyzed for total lactate content. It was found that the lactate concentration at exhaustion was higher in untrained muscle compared to trained muscle; therefore, the increased release in trained muscle can not be explained by a higher gradient, on the contrary the gradient from muscle to plasma was lower in trained muscle.

The improved release of lactate could also bee due to an increased content of lactate/H^+ co-transporter proteins called MCT1 and MCT4. To investigate this possibility, biopsy material from trained and untrained legs were analyzed for MCT content by western blotting (Figure 6).

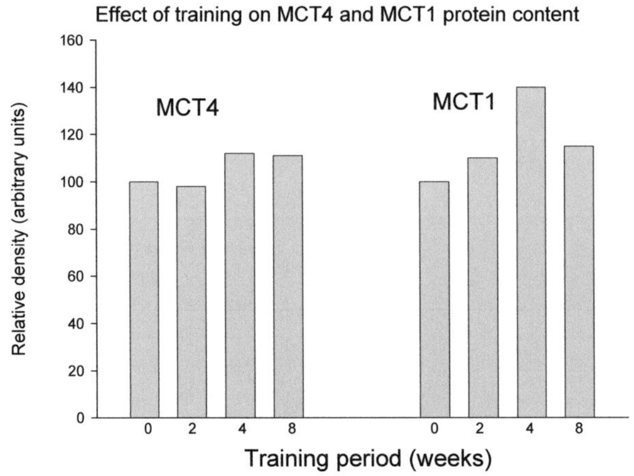

Fig. 6. Effects of 2, 4, and 8 weeks of high intensity training on muscle contents of the lactate/H^+ co-transporter proteins MCT4 and MCT1. Adapted from Juel et al. 2004)

Indeed, analyses of MCT content in biopsies obtained before, during and after the training period, demonstrated an increase in MCT content. However, the increase was moderate, and can only partly explain the dramatic increase in lactate release in the test experiments comparing trained and untrained leg (Figure 5). Could other mechanisms be involved?

Again biopsy material was used. The improved lactate release could be due to a higher blood flow in the trained compared to untrained muscle, which could be the underlying mechanism for a better wash-away of lactate, which maintains the gradient and facilitates a higher release. Biopsies were analyzed for number of capillaries per fiber (Jensen et al. 2004). The analysis demonstrated a considerable increase in the number of capillaries in the trained leg compared to untrained leg (Figure 7).

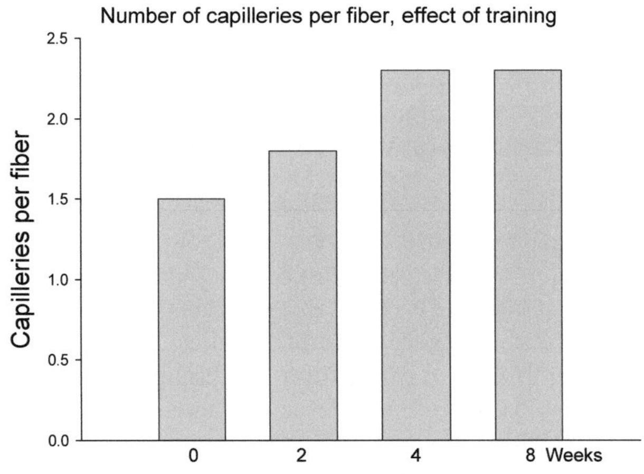

Fig. 7. Effect of training on number of capillaries per muscle fiber. Values determined in human biopsy material (data from Jensen et al. 2004).

Thus, the improvement in lactate release was partly due to a higher number of transporter molecules, and partly due to an improved blood flow. The improvement in blood flow was mainly mediated by an increased number of capillaries. In conclusion, analysis of biopsy material contributed with information about the underlying mechanisms.

3.2.3 Biopsies from patients

It is obvious that muscle biopsies are used for diagnostic purposes. Analyses of biopsy material can give information about cellular changes including metabolic changes. Analysis of pathological changes is outside the scope of the present review.

But biopsies have also been used for comparing patients and healthy control groups. One example is given below.

Diabetic patients and normal healthy control subjects differ in their insulin sensitivity and glucose handling. The use of biopsies has revealed other differences.

In a training study comparing diabetic patients and healthy control subjects it was found that type 2 diabetic patients had a lover muscle content of Na,K-pump subunits. For both groups strength training resulted in an increased density of pumps, but the diabetic patients still had a lover level of pump proteins (Dela et al. 2004). Likewise, studies of biopsy material from these groups demonstrated that type 2 diabetes is associated with a lower capacity for lactate and H^+ transport, and that the transport capacity could de increased with training in both groups (Juel et al. 2004a). In conclusion, type 2 diabetes is not only associated with reduced insulin sensitivity/reduced glucose transport, other membrane transport systems are also affected.

3.3 pH regulation in muscle

3.3.1 pH regulation in general

The concentration of H^+, which determines pH, is regulated by a number of mechanisms including several membrane transport system. The sum of all these mechanism is called pH regulation. The main problem in all living cells is that the negative membrane potential influences the distribution of H^+ across the outer membrane. The internal concentration of H^+ therefore tends to increase, and as a consequence there is a tendency towards a low intracellular pH (cellular acidification). The pH regulating system therefore has to remove free H^+ from the cell; this is either done by intracellular buffering or by transporting H^+ out (or OH^- in). For a review about pH regulation in human skeletal muscle see Juel (2008). The main components in pH regulation are outlined below.

3.3.2 Kinetics of pH regulation

Information about the kinetics of skeletal muscle pH regulation has been obtained both from whole body experiments and from experiments involving membrane vesicles.

3.3.3 Whole body experiments

Interstitial pH in human skeletal muscle can be measured with the microdialysis technique combined wit the use of pH sensitive dies (Street et al 2001). With this technique it has been possible to measure the time course of the pH changes associated with leg exercise with different intensities, see Figure 9.

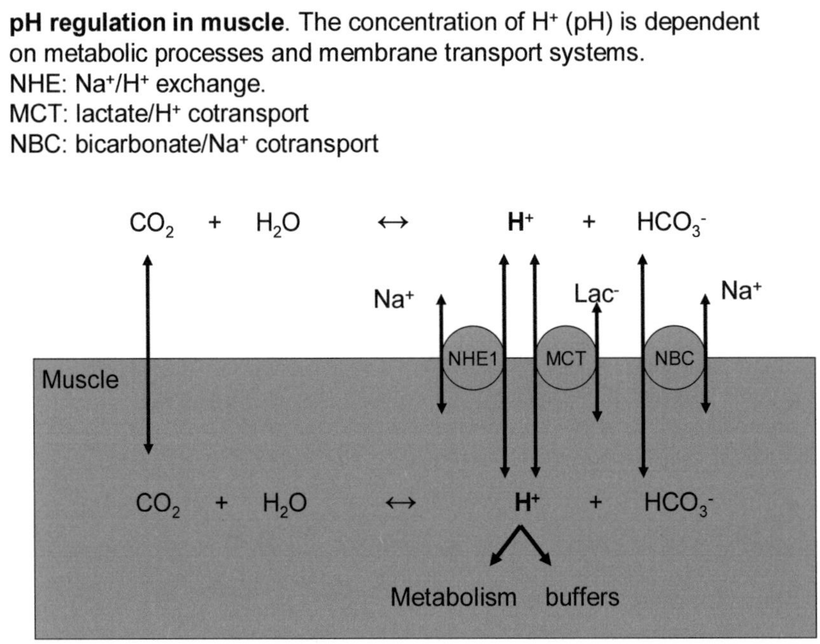

Fig. 8. Membrane transport proteins involved in pH regulation in skeletal muscle. Adapted from Juel et al. 2003.

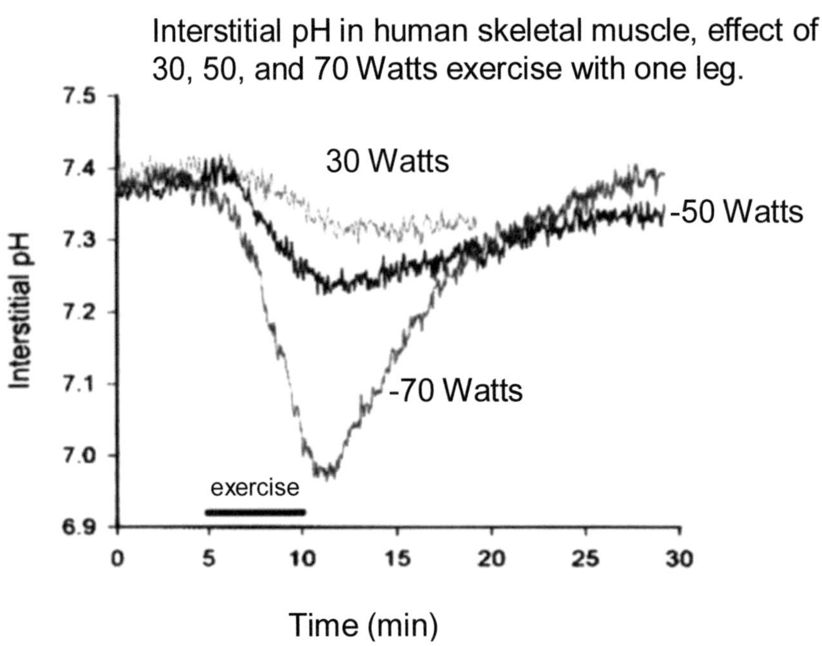

Fig. 9. Interstitial pH in human skeletal muscle during leg exercise with three different work intensities 30, 50 and 70 Watts. It can be seen that pH is reduced during exercise (acidification), and that recovery of pH takes place with a half-time of approximately 5 min. Data from Street et al. 2001.

3.3.4 Vesicle studies

Regulation of muscle pH has also been studied with sarcolemmal giant vesicles.

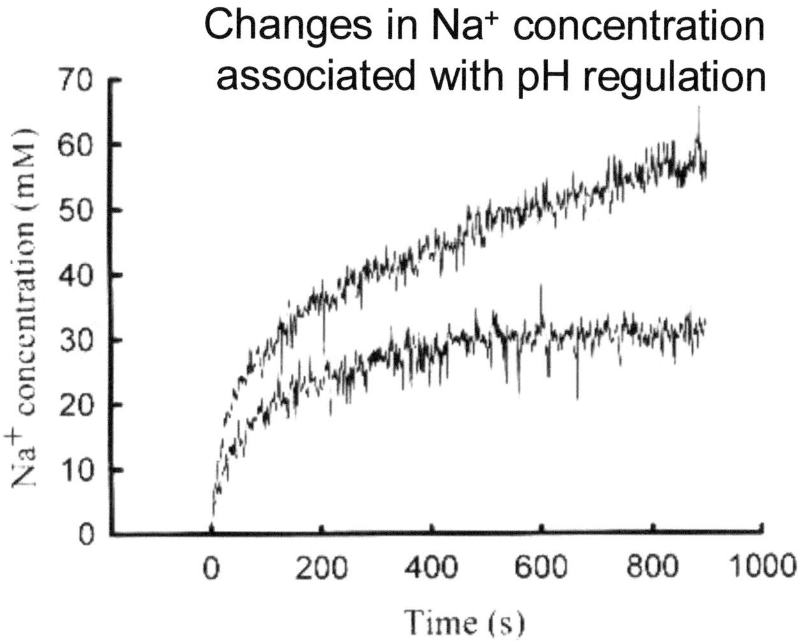

Fig. 10. pH regulation studied with vesicles obtained from rat skeletal muscle. At time zero external pH is changes 0.5 unit. Vesicular Na^+ concentration is measured with an ion sensitive dye. The changes in vesicular Na^+ concentration reveal that Na^+ fluxes across the membrane takes place during pH regulation. By the use of a specific inhibitor, amiloride, (lower trace) it was demonstrated that part of pH recovery is mediated by Na^+/H^+ exchange (Juel 2000).

3.3.5 The use of biopsy material to study other components of pH regulation

The sections below focus on the components involved in pH regulation.

3.3.6 Sodium/bicarbonate transport

Only a few studies have investigated the functional significance of sodium/bicarbonate co-transport in skeletal muscle in general and especially in human muscle. However, two isoforms of the Na^+/bicarbonate co-transporters NBCs have been identified in rat muscle and human muscle. For humans the experiments were based on biopsy material. Studies with vesicles made from rat have demonstrated that the NBCs contribution is approximately half of the total capacity for pH regulation in resting muscle (Kristensen et al. 2004).

3.3.7 Na^+/H^+ exchange

This exchanger is the classical pH regulating system found in most cell types. The kinetics of Na^+/H^+ exchange in skeletal muscle have been studied with rat muscle (Juel 1998, 1998,

2000). The effect of high-intensity training on human Na^+/H^+ exchange protein NHE1 has been studied with biopsy material obtained from trained and untrained muscle (Juel et al. 2004). Data from an animal study of Na^+/H^+ exchange in pH regulation is shown above, figure 10.

3.4 Ion homeostasis

Activation of skeletal muscle is associated with small displacements of ions; each action potential give rise to a small Na^+ influx and a small K^+ efflux due to opening if specific channel. During repeated activation Na^+ is accumulated in the muscle cell and K^+ is accumulated outside the cell. Analysis of blood samples obtained in association with muscle activity show an increased plasma K^+ concentration during muscle activity and in the first minute of the recovery period. The activity of the Na^+-K^+-pump counteracts these concentration changes, but it is obvious that the Na^+,K^+-pump can not keep pace with the K^+ efflux during muscle activity, which is the underlying mechanism for the extracellular accumulation of K^+ (Figure 11).

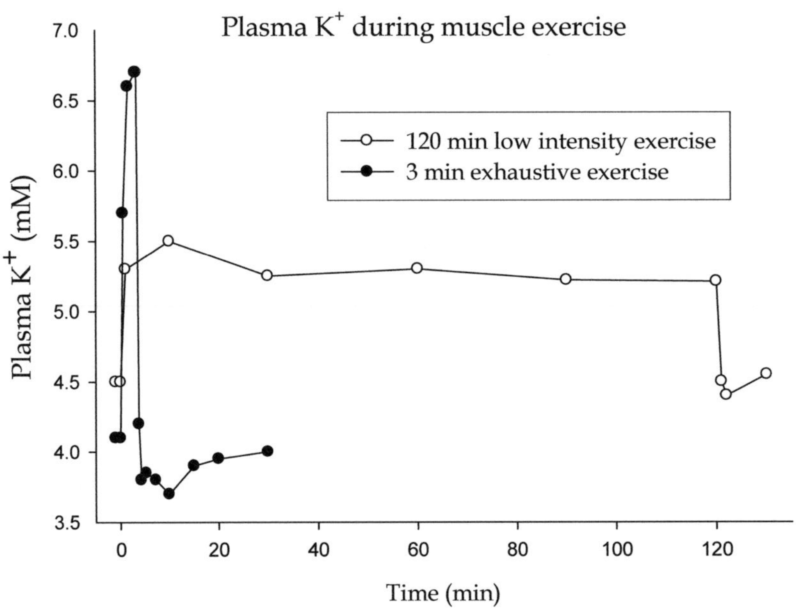

Fig. 11. Accumulation of K^+ in blood plasma during short intense muscle activity and during long lasting low intensity exercise. Potassium release was calculated from the arterial and venous blood K^+ concentration and blood flow. Data From Juel et al. 1990 and Sjøgaard 1986.

It can be concluded from Figure 11 that both short and long-lasting exercise is associated with a continuous potassium loss from muscle. It has been confirmed with muscle biopsies that the extracellular accumulation of K^+ is paralleled by a similar decrease in intracellular K^+ concentration.

The intracellular Na^+ increase and the extracellular K^+ concentration increase have been associated with muscle fatigue. The underlying mechanism is impaired muscle excitability, which results in reduced force; muscle fatigue. The Na^+,K^+-pump is the main membrane transport system responsible for ion homeostasis. The pump counteracts the ion displacements. Regulation of the pump is therefore important for development of fatigue. Stimulation of the pump by hormones and other mechanisms delays the development of fatigue.

3.4.1 Membrane purification, Western blotting

Analysis of sarcolemmal giant vesicle material with the use of specific membrane marker antibodies, has revealed that vesicular membranes exclusively consist of outer membranes with no contribution from T-tubuli and endoplasmatic reticulum membranes. This fact has been used in studies of protein distribution. The use of vesicles as a method to purify the outer membrane seems to be more efficient that the traditional methods, which include several spinning steps. This fact has been used to determine the cellular localization of membrane transport proteins, an example is given below.

3.4.2 Translocation of pumps

It was suggested before 2000, that the cell-surface Na,K-ATPase protein density in rat could be increased by insulin and exercise. But it was not known whether this mechanism is also present in human muscle. This was probably due to the large amount of muscle tissue needed for membrane purification. However, the development of the sarcolemmal giant vesicle technique and the optimization for the small amount of vesicles obtained from human muscle biopsies, made it possible to study the distribution of the Na,K-ATPase (Na,K-pump) in human skeletal muscle. In the first study to use this technique 6 human subjects performed one legged exercise until fatigue, and needle biopsies were obtained before exercise and immediately after fatigue. The amounts of Na,K-ATPase isoforms in the sarcolemmal membrane were measured with antibodies. It was demonstrated that exercise significantly increased the amount of $\alpha 2$, total α, and β subunit proteins by 70, 35 and 26 %, respectively (Juel et al. 2000). These values clearly indicated that pump subunits can be translocated from one store to the outer membrane during exercise. However, the underlying nature of this translocation remained unknown. It was later demonstrated with sarcolemmal material from rat muscle that the translocation of pump subunits to the outer membrane is reversible with a half-time of approximately 20 minutes (Juel et al. 2001).

The translocation mechanism has later been studied with other techniques including biotin labeling of surface membrane proteins in combination with sarcolemmal giant vesicles used as a membrane purification method (Kristensen et al. 2008). These studies confirmed that Na,K-ATPase subunits can translocate to the outer membrane. In addition it was demonstrated that changes in caveolae pump content could be part of the mechanism. This is another example of the use of biopsy material; these experiments clearly brought new knowledge.

3.4.3 Glucose transport

The use of sarcolemmal giant vesicles produced from biopsy material was a success in studies of lactate transport. It was therefore logic to use the same method for the study of glucose transport and glucose transporters. The first studies used vesicles from rat muscle. It was possible to demonstrate that glycose transport across the vesicular membranes was affected by insulin and muscle contractions (Ploug et al. 1993). Furthermore, the effect of pH and glucose-6-phosophate was studied (Kristiansen et al. 1994).

Studies of glucose transport using vesicles from human biopsies have also been published. Since vesicles exclusively consist of material from the outer membrane it is possible to investigate if the glucose transporters GLUT4 are translocated to the outer membrane during exercise. Changes in glucose transport and translocation of GLUT4 with endurance training have been investigated with vesicles produced from biopsies from human muscle (Richter et al. 1998) However, in spite of the first promising experiments with vesicles; this technique has not been used in newer experiments. The reason is that regulation of glucose transport is dependent on internal signaling pathways, which are lost during the preparation of vesicles.

3.4.4 Fri fatty acid transport

Long-chain fatty acids, LCFA, are important as an energy source in many tissues including skeletal muscle. It was originally believed that long chain-fatty acids can freely diffuse across the plasma membrane. It was early recognized that LCFA can bind to the outer membrane; the binding proteins were simply called fatty acid binding proteins. The details could only be studied in a model system; again vesicles were used. The early studies of fatty acid membrane transport were carried out with sarcolemmal giant vesicles produced from rat muscle (Bonen et al, 1999; Luiken et al., 2001; Turcotte at al., 2000; Bonen et al., 1998; Bonen et al., 2000). It was demonstrated that the transport showed saturation and could be inhibited with specific antibodies, which clearly indicates that a transport system is involved (Turcotte et al. 2000).

These studies in combination with the use of antibodies and western blotting revealed three groups of transport systems: fatty acid binding proteins (FABPm), fatty acid translocase (FAT), and fatty acid transporter proteins (FATP)(Bonen et al. 1998a). These early transport studies were not based on human membrane material. But human biopsy material was later used to identify the transporter proteins in human skeletal muscle (Roepstorff et al. 2004). In addition, biopsies taken before and after training were used to characterize the effect of endurance training on the FABPm protein density, which was increased by 49 % after three weeks of training (Kiens et al. 1997).

4. Conclusion

Whole body experiments in humans have given much information about membrane transport. These data have been combined with information obtained by the use of biopsies.

Biopsies from human skeletal muscle have been used to give a snapshot of metabolite content and ion composition in connection with muscle activity and training. It is also possible to study dynamic aspects of gene regulation in human biopsy material.

The present review has focused on studies of membrane transport based on biopsy material. It has been shown that muscle treated with collagenase and high K^+ concentrations induce formation of membrane vesicles. Single vesicles were originally used for microelectrode recordings of ion currents (Burton et al. 1990). A method to purification vesicles made from animal muscle was later developed (Juel 1990), and the method was further developed allowing vesicles to be produced from human skeletal muscle biopsies (Juel et al. 1994). These vesicles were demonstrated to be a new and unique method to investigate membrane transport processes in human skeletal muscle. In combination with the use of radio-labeled tracers these vesicles allowed quantification of the transport kinetic parameters K_m and V_{max} (per square cm of membrane).

The first membrane transport system to be investigated in humans with the biopsy based vesicle technique was the lactate/proton co-transport system. This transport system was characterized first in rat skeletal muscle membranes later in membranes from human skeletal muscle (Juel 1991, Pilegaard et al. 1993, Juel et al. 1994). With this technique it was possible to measure lactate/proton co-transport in muscle fiber types and to show that this transport system could be up-regulated with training and decreased with inactivity. It must be noted that the first discovered adaptive changes was quantified before the transport protein was cloned and before antibodies were available. Later studies have used vesicles as a method to purify muscle membranes. These studies were combined with information obtained by whole body experiments.

Sarcolemmal giant vesicles have later been used to study:

- glucose transport (Kristiansen et al. 1994)
- pH regulation (Juel 1995)
- translocation of Na,K-pump subunits (Juel et al. 2001)
- Na^+/H^+ exchange
- K^+ displacement during exercise
- membrane transport of free fatty acids (Bonen et al. 1998)

Data from biopsies were also used in exercise and training experiments. These studies gained from the fact that a biopsy represents a snapshoot of the metabolic and ionic content of an active muscle.

5. References

Bergström, J. (1962). Muscle electrolytes in man. Determined by neutron activation analyses of needle biopsy specimens. A study on normal subjects, kidney patients and patients with chronic diarrhoea. *Scand J Clin Lab Invest* vol.14, pp. 1-110.

Bonen, A.; Luiken, J.J.; Liu, S.; Dyck, D.J.; Kiens, B.; Kristiansen, S.; Turcotte, L.P.; Van der Vusse, G.J. & Glatz, J.F. (1998) . Palmitate transport and fatty acid transporters in red and white muscles. *Am J Physiol, Vol.*275, No 3 Pt 1, pp. E471-E478

Bonen, A.; Dyck, D.J.; Ibrahimi, A. & Abumrad, N.A. (1999). Muscle contractile activity increases fatty acid metabolism and transport and FAT/CD36. *Am J Physiol* Vol.276 pp. E643-9

Bonen, A.; Dyck, D.J. & Luiken, J.J. (1998). Skeletal muscle fatty acid transport and transporters. *Adv Exp Med Biol.* Vol. 441 pp. 193-205.

Bonen, A.; Joost, J.F.P.; Luiken, J.; Arumugam,Y.; Glatz, J.F.C. & Tandon, N.N. (2000). Acute regulation of fatty acid uptake involves the cellular redistribution of fatty acid translocase. *J Biol Chem*, Vol. 275 pp. 14501-14508

Burton, F.L. & Hutter, O.F. (1990). Sensitivity to flow of intrinsic gating in inward rectifying potassium channels from mammalian skeletal muscle. *J Physiol* Vol. 424, pp. 253-261.

Dela, F.; Holten, M. & Juel, C. (2004). Effect of resistance training on Na,K pump and Na^+/H^+ exchange protein densities in muscle from control and patients with type 2 diabetes. *Pflügers Arch – Eur J Physiol* Vol. 447 pp. 928-933.

Hildebrand, A.L. & Neufer, P.D. (2000). Exercise attenuates the fasting-induced transcriptional activation of metabolic genes in skeletal muscle. *Am J Physiol Endocrinol Metab* Vol. 278 pp. E1078-86

Jensen, L.; Bangsbo. J. & Hellsten, Y. (2004). Effect of high intensity training on capillarization and presence of angiogenic factors in human skeletal muscle. *J Physiol* Vol. 557 pp. 571-582.

Juel, C. (1991). Muscle lactate transport studied in sarcolemmal giant vesicles. *Biochim Biophys Acta Vol.* 1065, pp. 15-20.

Juel, C. (1995). Regulation of cellular pH in skeletal muscle fiber types, studied with sarcolemmal giant vesicles obtained from rat muscles. *Biochim Biophys Acta* Vol.1265, pp. 127-132.

Juel, C. (1998). Skeletal muscle Na^+/H^+ exchange in rats: pH dependency and the effect of training. *Acta Physiol Scand* Vol. 164, pp. 135-140

Juel, C. (1998). Muscle pH regulation: role of training. *Acta Physiol Scand* Vol. 162, pp. 350-366.

Juel, C. (2000). Expression of the Na^+/H^+ exchanger isoform NHE1 in rat skeletal muscle. *Acta Physiol Scand* Vol. 170 pp. 59-63.

Juel, C. (2006). Training-induced changes in membrane transport proteins of human skeletal muscle. *Eur J Appl Physiol* Vol. 96, pp. 627-635.

Juel, C. (2008). Regulation of pH in human skeletal muscle: adaptations to physical activity. *Acta Physiol Scand* Vol. 193, pp. 17-24.

Juel, C.; Bangsbo, J.; Graham, T. & Saltin, B. (1990). Lactate and potassium fluxes from human skeletal muscle during and after intense, dynamic, knee extensor exercise. *Acta Physiol Scand* Vol.140 pp. 147-159.

Juel, C.; Grunnet, L.; Holse, M.; Kenworthy, S.; Sommer, V. & Wulff, T. (2001). Reversibility of exercise- induced translocation of Na^+-K^+ pump subunits to the plasma membrane in rat skeletal muscle. *Pflügers Arch- Eur J Physiol* Vol. 443 pp.: 212-217.

Juel, C.; Holten, M.K. & Dela, F. (2004a). Effect of strength training on muscle lactate release and MCT1 and MCT4 content in healthy and type 2 diabetic humans. *J Physiol* Vol. 556 pp. 297-304.

Juel, C.; Klarskov, C.; Nielsen, J.J.; Krustrup, P.; Mohr, M. & Bangsbo, J. (2004). Effect of high-intensity intermittent training on lactate and H^+ release from human skeletal muscle. *Am J Physiol Endocrinol Metab* Vol. 286, pp. E245-E251.

Juel, C.; Kristiansen, S.; Pilegaard, H.; Wojtaszewski, J. & Richter, E.A. (1994). Kinetics of Lactate Transport in Sarcolemmal Giant Vesicles Obtained from Human Skeletal Muscle. *J Appl Physiol* Vol. 76, pp. 1031-1036.

Juel, C.; Lundby, C.; Sander, M.; Calbet, J.A.L. & Hall, G.V. (2003). Human skeletal muscle and erythrocyte proteins involved in acid-base homeostasis: adaptations to chronic hypoxia. *J Physiol* Vol. 548 pp. 639-648.

Juel, C.; Nielsen, J.J. & Bangsbo, J. (2000). Exercise-induced translocation of Na^+-K^+ pump subunits to the plasma membrane in human skeletal muscle. *Am J Physiol Reg Int Comp Physiol* Vol. 278, pp. R1107-R1110.

Kiens, B.; Kristiansen, S.; Jensen, P.; Richter, E.A. & Turcotte, L.P. (1997). Membrane associated fatty acid binding proteins (FABPm) in human skeletal muscle is increased by endurance training. *Biochem Biophys Res Commun* Vol. 231, pp. 463-465.

Kristensen, J.M.; Kristensen, M.; & Juel, C. (2004). Expression of Na^+/HCO_3^- co-transporter proteins (NBCs) in rat and human skeletal muscle. *Acta Physiol Scand* Vol.182, pp. 69-76.

Kristensen, M.; Rasmussen, M.K. & Juel, C. (2008). Na^+-K^+ pump location and translocation during muscle contraction in rat skeletal muscle. *Pflügers Arch – Eur J Physiol* Vol.456, pp. 979-989.

Kristiansen, S.; Wojtaszewski, J.F.; Juel, C. & Richter, E.A. (1994). Effect of glucose-6-phosphate and pH on glucose transport in skeletal muscle plasma membrane giant vesicles. *Acta Physiol Scand* Vol.150, pp. 227-233.

Luiken, J.J.; Arumugam, Y.; Dyck, D.J.; Bell, R.C.; Pelsers, M.M.; Turcotte, L.P.; Tandon, N.N.; Glatz, J.F. & Bonen, A. (2001). Increased rate of fatty acid uptake and plasmalemmal fatty acid transporters in obese Zucker rats. *J Biol Chem* Vol.276, pp. 40567-73.

Ploug, T.; Wojtaszewski, J.; Kristiansen, S.; Hespel, P.; Galbo, H. & Richter, E.A. (1993). Glucose transport and transporters in muscle giant vesicles: differential effect of insulin and contractions. *Am J Physiol* Vol. 264, pp. E270-E278.

Pilegaard, H.; Bangsbo, J.; Richter, E.A. & Juel, C. (1994). Lactate transport studied in sarcolemmal giant vesicles from human muscle biopsies - relation to training status. *J Appl Physiol* Vol.77, pp. 1858-1862.

Pilegaard, H.; Domino, K.; Noland, T.; Juel, C.; Hellsten, Y.; Halestrap, A.P. & Bangsbo, J. (1999). Effect of high-intensity exercise training on lactate/H^+ transport capacity in human skeletal muscle. *Am J Physiol Endocrinol Metab* Vol. 276, pp. E225-E261.

Pilegaard, H; Ordway, G.A.; Saltin, B. & Neufer, P.D. (2000). Transcriptional regulation of gene expression in human skeletal muscle during recovery from exercise. *Am J Physiol Endocrinol Metab* Vol. 279, pp. E806-E814.

Richter, E.A.; Jensen, P.; Kiens, B. & Kristiansen, S. (1998). Sarcolemmal glucose transport and GLUT-4 translocation during exercise are diminished by endurance training. *Am J Physiol* Vol. 274, pp. E89-E95.

Roepstorff, C.; Helge, J.W.; Vistisen, B. & Kiens, B. (2004). Studies of plasma membrane fatty acid-binding protein and other lipid binding proteins in human skeletal muscle. *Proc Nutr Soc* Vol. 63, pp. 239-244.

Sjøgaard, G. (1986). Water and electrolyte fluxes during exercise and their relation to muscle fatigue. *Acta Physiol Scand.* Vol. 128, pp. 129-136

Street, D.; Bangsbo, J & Juel, C. (2001). Interstitial pH in human skeletal muscle during and after dynamic graded exercise. *J Physiol* Vol. 537, pp. 993-998.

Turcotte, L.P.; Swenberger, J.R.; Tucker, M.Z.; Yee, A.J.; Trump, G.; Luiken, J.J. & Bonen, A. (2000). Muscle palmitate uptake and binding are saturable and inhibited by antibodies to FABP(PM). *Mol Cell Biochem* Vol. 210, pp. 53-63.

Wilson, M.C.; Jackson, V.N.; Heddie, C.; Price, N.T.; Pilegaard, H.; Juel, C.; Bonen, A.; Montgommery, I.; Hutter, O.F. & Halestrap, A.P. (1998). Lactic acid efflux from white skeletal muscle is catalysed by the monocarboxylate transporter MCT3. *J Biol Chem* Vol. 273, pp. 15920-15926.

Part 3

Muscle Biopsy: Metabolic Diseases

5

Evaluation of Mitochondrial Functions and Dysfunctions in Muscle Biopsy Samples

Frédéric Capel[1,2], Valentin Barquissau[1,2], Ruddy Richard[1,2] and Béatrice Morio[1,2]
[1]*INRA, UMR1019 Nutrition Humaine, CRNH Auvergne, F-63120 Saint-Genès-Champanelle*
[2]*Université Clermont 1, UMR1019 Nutrition Humaine, UFR Medicine, F-63000 Clermont-Ferrand*
France

1. Introduction

Within the past decade, the list of publications involving mitochondrial dysfunction in the etiology of metabolic disorders in obesity, insulin resistance and type 2 diabetes, has been growing steadily. Today, large controversies still exist and it is clear that the understanding of the causes and consequences of impairments in mitochondrial functioning are far from being accomplished. In this context, our purpose is to review techniques used in human samples to highlight defects in mitochondrial activity, with a particular focus on skeletal muscle. Several tools are described to assess a large array of mitochondrial functions. In order to facilitate the reading of the review, several details related to methodological concerns are provided in supplementary materials and remain available upon request to the authors.

2. Basic knowledge on mitochondrial functioning

Mitochondria are found in nearly all eukaryotes. They are forming a complex network which shape and functioning is determined by the interaction with the cytoskeleton and by the balance between fusion and fission reactions (Zorzano et al., 2009). They vary in number and location according to cell type. Within skeletal muscle fibers, mitochondrial density and activity mainly varies according to fiber types and physical training (Howald et al., 1985) although type 2 diabetes and genetic inheritance have been also proposed as potential modulators (Petersen et al., 2004; Morio et al., 2005; Befroy et al., 2007). Mitochondria are located either around the nuclei, this subgroup is called subsarcolemmal mitochondria, or nestled between myofibrils. These mitochondria are named intermyofibrillar and have distinct activity from subsarcolemmal ones (Koves et al., 2005; Mollica et al., 2006). Intermyofibrillar mitochondria are mainly dedicated to energy production for muscle fiber contraction. By contrast, subsarcolemmal mitochondria may play a key role in signal transduction and substrate transport. Deficiency in the latter pool has been proposed to contribute to the pathogenesis of muscle insulin resistance in type 2 diabetes (Ritov et al., 2005; Benton et al., 2008).

The most prominent role of mitochondria is to produce the "energy carrier" adenosine triphosphate (ATP) mainly from glucose and fatty acid oxidation, and to a lesser extend from amino acid oxidation. Nutrient oxidation within the cytosol and/or the mitochondrial matrix results in acetyl-CoA production, the main substrate of the tricarboxylic acid (TCA) cycle which takes place in the mitochondrial matrix. The β-oxidation pathway is specific to fatty acid oxidation and results in acetyl-CoA production which feeds TCA cycle. These oxidative pathways are coupled to the mitochondrial electron transport chain (ETC), whose enzyme content and activity together define the mitochondrial oxidative capacity. The latter factor combined with mitochondrial density determines the tissue oxidative capacity. The main rate-limiting oxidative enzymes are citrate synthase and isocitrate dehydrogenase (TCA cycle), β-hydroxyacyl-CoA dehydrogenase (β-oxidation) and cytochrome c oxidase (ETC). Mitochondria are also key organelles for regulation of cell metabolism. Mitochondrial functioning has been proven to control cellular metabolism, redox and calcium signalling, apoptosis-programmed cell death and cellular proliferation. This shows that a perpetual cross talk exists between cell and mitochondria, the result being the cell adaptation to physiological changes or the cell death (Figure 1).

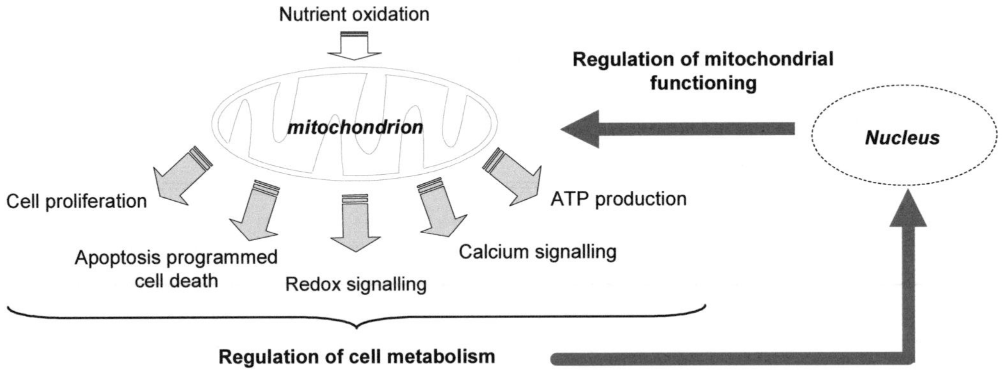

Fig. 1. Involvement of the cross-talk between nucleus and mitochondria in the regulation of cell adaptations.

2.1 Mitochondrial respiratory chain, membrane potential and energy production, and main alterations observed in metabolic disorders

Nutrient oxidation consists in a series of enzyme-catalysed oxidative reactions which aims at transferring energy-rich electrons to the cofactors nicotinamide adenine dinucleotide [NAD+] and flavin mononucleotide [FAD], forming respectively NADH, H^+ and $FADH_2$. The latter reduced carriers provide thereafter the ETC with these energy-rich electrons. The ETC is situated into the mitochondrial inner membrane and consists of four large enzyme complexes (Complex I, NADH-CoQ oxidoreductase; II, succinate dehydrogenase; III, CoQ-cytochrome c oxidoreductase; and IV, cytochrome c oxidase). Mobile electron carriers (e.g. coenzyme Q or ubiquinone, and cytochrome c) transport the electrons from one complex to the next with oxygen acting as the final electron acceptor within cytochrome c oxidase. The transfer of the high-energy electrons along the electron transport chain results in the pumping of H^+ ions across the inner membrane, creating an electrochemical gradient (also named membrane potential, $\Delta\psi m$) that provides the energy required to drive the synthesis of ATP thanks to a fifth complex called F_0F_1 ATP synthase. The latter consists of a H^+ ion channel (F_0) connected to a catalytic subunit (F_1). The energy provided by the flux of H^+ ions through F_0 is used to drive ATP synthesis from ADP and Pi by F_1 (Figure 2). The electrochemical gradient determines the coupling between the oxidative and the phosphorylative reactions. It is named oxidative phosphorylation (OXPHOS).

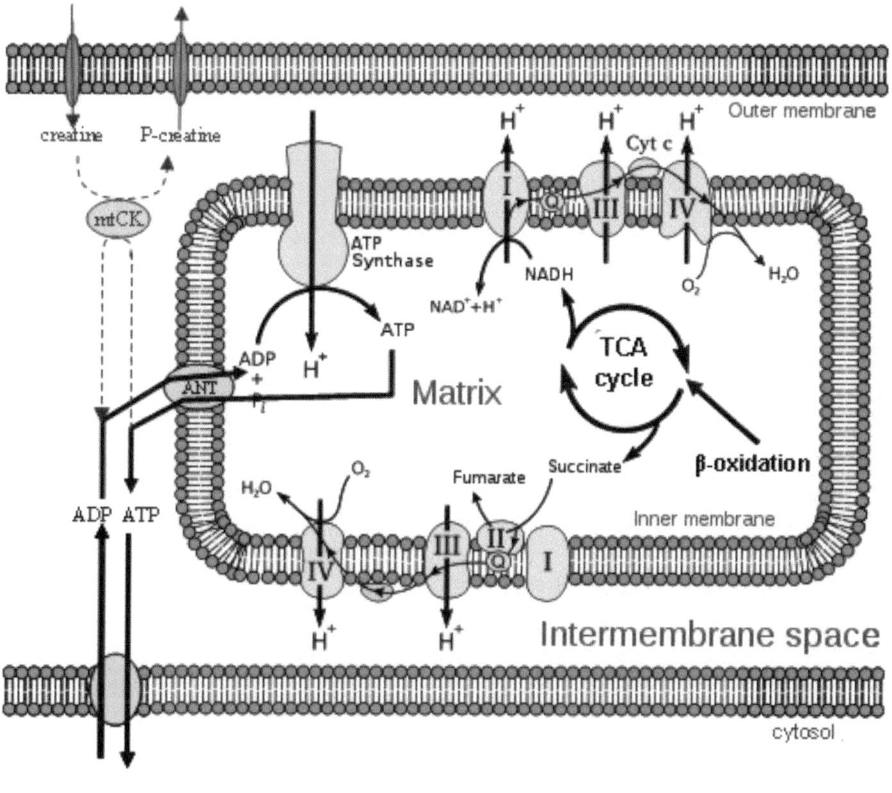

Fig. 2. Main organization of mitochondrial oxidative and phosphorylative pathways. TCA cycle, tricarboxylic cycle; Complex I, NADH-CoQ oxidoreductase; Complex II, succinate dehydrogenase; Complex III, CoQ-cytochrome c oxidoreductase; Complex IV, cytochrome c oxidase; Q, coenzyme Q or ubiquinone; Cyt c, cytochrome c; ANT, adenine nucleotide translocase, ANT; mtCK, creatine kinase. *This figure is derived from Wikipedia.*

Mitochondrial membrane potential is a key indicator of cellular viability. As demonstrated by Peter Mitchell (1961), it is the driving force behind ATP production. It also governs ROS production, mitochondrial calcium storage, opening of mitochondrial permeability transition pores (mPTP) and mitochondrial-apoptotic programmed cell death (reviews in Casteilla et al., 2001; Hand & Menze, 2008). Mitochondrial ATP production has to strictly match cellular needs. It is tightly controlled by different factors. The ATP/ADP-Pi ratio, through a mitochondrial ADP sensing which is still not fully understood (Wilson et al., 1977), the NAD+/NADH-H+ ratio and local oxygen pressure chance. The transfers of ATP, ADP and Pi between the cytosol and the mitochondrial matrix involve ATP/ADP carriers (adenine nucleotide translocase, ANT). The high-energy phosphate group of ATP may be also transferred to creatine to yield phosphocreatine. This reaction is catalyzed by the mitochondrial isoform of creatine kinase (mtCK), which is located in the mitochondrial intermembrane space. The dynamic of the phosphate group transfer between ATP and creatine and the transport of these metabolites between cytosol and mitochondrial intermembrane space, differs between contractile fiber types. This is due to differential coupling between mtCK, ANT and porin (voltage-dependent anion channel, VDAC) which determines the flux of ADP entrance within the mitochondrial matrix (Saks et al., 1994). Unlike glycolytic fibers (type IIb) for which mitochondrial respiration is regulated by cytosolic ADP, mitochondrial respiration of oxidative fibers (type I) is more controlled by the ratio between creatine and phosphocreatine than by ADP (Zoll et al., 2003). The oxydo-glycolytic fibers (type IIa) present an intermediate situation.

Except in Asian Indians, consistent decrease in muscle mitochondrial ATP production has been reported in insulin resistance in obesity and type 2 diabetes (Petersen et al., 2004, 2005; Szendroedi et al., 2007; Chanseaume et al., 2010). By contrast, the theory linking insulin resistance to decreased mitochondrial oxidative capacity is more challenged. It has been supported by several cross-sectional studies in obese insulin-resistant and type 2 diabetic patients compared to healthy individuals (Howald et al., 1985; Kelley et al., 2002; Pertersen et al., 2004; Ritov et al., 2005, 2010). These observational studies are reviewed in table 1. By contrast, recent studies (Petersen et al., 2005; Chanseaume et al., 2010) and clinical trials that involve interventions (weight loss, physical activity) altering insulin sensitivity (Brons et al., 2008; Toledo et al., 2008) demonstrated a dissociation between insulin resistance and mitochondrial functioning in skeletal muscle. Part of the discrepancy may be due to bias induced by confounding factors, such as physical activity. Indeed when the latter factor is rigorously taken into account, mitochondrial oxidative capacity is similar between lean and obese-insulin resistant volunteers (Chanseaume et al., 2010). However, genetic and/or epigenetic predisposition have also to be taken into account (Petersen et al., 2004, 2005; Morino et al., 2005; Befroy et al., 2007; Nair et al., 2008).

2.2 Mitochondrial fatty acid oxidation and cellular meanings

Mitochondria are the principal site of long-chain fatty acid (LCFA) oxidation for cellular energy production. A defect in this process may trigger the accumulation of toxic lipid metabolites in skeletal muscle. Mitochondrial LCFA oxidation is tightly regulated by the enzyme carnitine palmitoyltransferase 1 (CPT1), which is situated in the outer mitochondrial membrane and regulates the entry of acyl-CoAs into mitochondria. Malonyl-CoA, the first metabolic intermediate of lipogenesis produced by the enzyme acetyl-CoA carboxylase, is the physiological allosteric inhibitor of CPT1 (McGarry & Brown, 1997). This malonyl-CoA/CPT1 partnership is considered as a "fuel sensor" whose role is to regulate the rate of LCFA oxidation according to the relative disposal of LCFA and glucose within the cell. When circulating lipids increase, whereas glucose availability decreases (such as during starvation), lipids are oxidized in mitochondria at the expense of glucose (Rasmussen & Wolfe, 1999). When mitochondrial LCFA oxidative capacity becomes limited, excess LCFAs taken up by the cell are initially redirected towards storage in the form of triacylglycerols (TAG). For these reasons, new concept has emerged pointing out muscle mitochondrial dysfunction as the leading cause for TAG accumulation in obesity and insulin resistance (Petersen & Shulman, 2006).

Measured parameters	Population studied	Results	References
Mitochondrial content	Insulin resistant with family predisposition	?	Morino et al., 2005
	Obese	?	Holloway et al., 2007
	Obese and insulin resistant*	=	Chanseaume et al., 2010
	Obese and type-2 diabetic	?	Ritov et al., 2005
	Type-2 diabetic	?	Boushel et al., 2007
	Type-2 diabetic	=	Nair et al., 2008
	Type-2 diabetic	=	Ashmann et al., 2006
Morphology	Obese and type-2 diabetic	? size, area	Kelley et al., 2002
	Type-2 diabetic	? size	Ritov et al., 2005
Biogenesis signalling pathway	Insulin resistant with family predisposition	? PGC-1a, complexes 1-3-4	Heilbronn et al., 2007
	Insulin resistant with family predisposition	= PGC-1a, OXPHOS	Brons et al., 2008
	Obese and insulin resistant*	= PGC-1a/ß, NRF1, OXPHOS	Chanseaume et al., 2010
	Type-2 diabetic and insulin resistant with predisposition	? PGC-1a/ß, NRF1, OXPHOS	Patti et al., 2003
	Type-2 diabetic	? PGC-1a/ß, OXPHOS	Mootha et al., 2003
	Type-2 diabetic	? PGC-1a	Debard et al., 2004
	Type-2 diabetic	= PGC-1a/ß, NRF1, OXPHOS	Nair et al., 2008
Substrates oxidation	Obese	? LCFA oxidation	Kim et al., 2000
	Insulin resistant with family predisposition	? acetyl-CoA oxidation	Befroy et al., 2007
Maximal enzyme activity	Insulin resistant	? Citrate synthase	Heilbronn et al., 2007
	Obese	? CPT1, ßHAD, citrate synthase	Kim et al., 2000
	Obese	? CPT1, ßHAD, COX	Holloway et al., 2007
	Obese and insulin resistant*	= Citrate synthase, COX	Chanseaume et al., 2010
	Obese and type-2 diabetic	? Complexe 2	Ritov et al., 2005
	Obese and type-2 diabetic	? Complexe 2	He et al., 2001
	Obese and type-2 diabetic	? Citrate synthase, complexe 1	Kelley et al., 2002
	Type-2 diabetic	? Citrate synthase	Boushel et al., 2007
	Type-2 diabetic	? Citrate synthase	Ortenblad et al., 2005
	Type-2 diabetic	= Citrate synthase	Nair et al., 2008
ATP synthesis	Insulin resistant with family predisposition	?	Petersen et al., 2004
	Insulin resistant with family predisposition	?	Petersen et al., 2005
	Obese and insulin resistant*	?	Chanseaume et al., 2010
	Obese and type-2 diabetic	?	Abdul-Ghani et al., 2009
	Type-2 diabetic	?	Szendroedi et al., 2007
	Type-2 diabetic	=	Nair et al., 2008
P-creatine synthesis	Insulin resistant with predisposition	=	Brons et al., 2008
	Type-2 diabetic	?	Schrauwen-Hinderling et al., 2007
ROS production	Obese and insulin resistant*	?	Chanseaume et al., 2010
	Obese and type-2 diabetic	? in obese, = in type-2 diabetic	Abdul-Ghani et al., 2009

Table 1. Alterations in mitochondrial structure, content and functioning reported in skeletal muscle of insulin resistant, obese and/or type-2 diabetic patients. * all volunteers were similarly sedentary

Cellular TAG buffering capacity in lean tissues such as skeletal muscle, is limited and rapidly flooded, especially for saturated LCFAs such as palmitate which are poorly incorporated into TAG (garcia-Martinez et al., 2005). In these conditions, excess LCFAs may enter alternative non-oxidative pathways that result in the production and accumulation of toxic lipid metabolites, such as diacylglycerols (DAG), acyl-CoAs or ceramides. These LCFA derivatives have been demonstrated to be deleterious for cell functioning since they are able to modulate activity of protein kinases (Shulman, 2000; Hegarty et al., 2003) which ultimately trigger insulin resistance (Shulman, 2000; Chavez et al., 2005), mitochondrial dysfunction (Coll et al., 2006), oxidative stress (Montuschi et al., 2004) and apoptosis (Slawik & Vidal-Puig, 2006). Whereas mechanisms linking those LCFA metabolites to insulin resistance have raised large consensus, the involvement of mitochondrial LCFA oxidative capacity in the regulation of their synthesis rates is still controversial (Rimbert et al., 2004, 2009). These arguments suggest that more complex interactions exist between LCFA availability and cell metabolism, and determine the intracellular fates of LCFAs (for review Kewalramani et al., 2010).

2.3 Mitochondrial production of reactive oxygen species and cell consequences

During the electron transfer through the respiratory chain, a small percentage of electrons may prematurely reduce oxygen, forming reactive oxygen species (ROS) such as superoxide anion radicals ($O_2^{\bullet -}$). It was demonstrated that the main sites of ROS production are located at complexes I and III, the iron-sulphur centers of complex I being potentially the most important ROS generators (Barja, 1999). ROS are generated either from "normal" electron transfer after oxidation of substrates of complex I and complex II, but also from "reversed" electron transfer from complex II towards complex I (Liu et al., 2002). The latter situation is suggested to be the most physiologically relevant ROS production in mammals (Miwa & Brand, 2003). Recent work from Seifert et al. (2010) showed that LCFA β-oxidation is associated with enhanced ROS production, through a mechanism involving complex III, the electron transfer flavoprotein (ETF) and ETF-oxidoreductase.

As reviewed by Murphy (2009), the rate of ROS production is mainly determined by the membrane potential, the ratio between NADH and NAD+, the ratio between CoQH2 and CoQ and the local O_2 concentration. It is well established that there is a strong positive correlation between membrane potential and ROS production. Small increase in membrane potential has been associated to a large stimulation of ROS production (Korshunov et al., 1997). Similarly, a small decrease in membrane potential deeply reduces ROS production (Votyakova & Reynolds, 2001). Therefore mild uncoupling resulting from a small decrease in membrane potential is considered as a natural antioxidant process (Seifert et al., 2010; Skulachev, 1997). However, not all sites of ROS production are sensitive to membrane potential. Indeed, Seifert et al. (2010) found that the ROS produced during LCFA β-oxidation and involving complex III, ETF and ETF-oxidoreductase, was relatively insensitive to membrane potential changes. In addition, Miwa and Brand reported that the ROS produced at the cytosolic side of complex I through glycerol-3-phosphate dehydrogenase, which donates electrons to the electron carrier Q, is insensitive to membrane potential (2003). By contrast, ROS production from complex I following reverse electron flow is highly sensitive to membrane potential. Mild uncoupling is based on a proton leak across the inner membrane. It is mediated by thyroid hormones, LCFAs, complex IV slipping but most importantly by the activity of the uncoupling proteins UCP2 and UCP3, although molecular mechanism are still not well understood (for review see Murphy, 2009; Schrauwen & Hesselink, 2002; Bezaire et al., 2007). Whereas overexpression of UCP in skeletal muscle has been shown to prevent diet-induced obesity and insulin resistance in mice (Li et al., 2000), their specific involvement in mitochondrial functioning and muscle metabolism in obesity and type 2 diabetes is still under debate in humans (Krook et al., 1998; Bao et al., 1998; Samec et al., 1999).

Spontaneously or by the action of superoxide dismutase (SOD), $O_2^{\bullet -}$ dismutates into hydrogen peroxide H_2O_2, which is more stable and can diffuse through biological membranes. H_2O_2 has been shown to inhibit TCA cycle oxidative enzymes (alpha-ketoglutarate dehydrogenase, succinate dehydrogenase, aconitase) and complex II (Moser et al., 2009; Nulton-Persson & Szweda, 2001). It is an important signal molecule, regulating major redox signalling pathways (for review see Leloup et al., 2011). It can also react to form hydroxyl radical or peroxynitrite, which are both highly damaging. In that context, oxidative stress can occur due to the accumulation of oxidative damages within DNA, protein and lipid components of the organelle. This may contribute to the decline in mitochondrial function and lead in turn to enhanced ROS generation. This vicious circle has been involved in many pathologies and the aging process. It is however questioned in the aetiology of insulin resistance in obesity and type 2 diabetes because reduced mitochondrial ROS production has been reported in those latter situations (Abdul-Ghani et al., 2009; Chanseaume & Morio, 2009). Because mitochondrial dysfunction in type 2 diabetes has been related to oxidative stress (Bonnard et al., 2008), other cellular sites of ROS production are potentially involved.

2.4 Mitochondrial calcium storage and cellular consequences

Mitochondrial calcium uptake has been first described in the early 1960s (Deluca & Engstrom, 1961; Vasington & Murphy, 1962). Since then it has been recognized that mitochondria are able to store amount of calcium bound to phosphate within their matrix large (review in Nicholls & Chalmers, 2004). Differential regulation of mitochondrial Ca^{2+} uptake and release are presented by Hoppe (2010). Calcium taken up by the mitochondria regulates mitochondrial functioning in response to a variety of extracellular stimuli (Jouaville et al., 1999; Territo et al., 2000). It activates three dehydrogenases of the TCA cycle, pyruvate dehydrogenase, isocitrate dehydrogenase, and α-keto glutarate dehydrogenase (63). It may also regulate the ETC, the F_0F_1ATP synthase and ANT (McCormack et al., 1990). This induces an increased substrate uptake by mitochondria, enhanced mitochondrial NADH/NAD^+ ratio and increased ATP production. The high capacity to accumulate calcium confer to mitochondria a key role in the regulation of intracellular calcium signalling (Gunter KK & Gunter TE, 1994; Rizzuto et al., 1998), which includes regulation of gene expression (including those involved in mitochondrial biogenesis and glucose uptake), cell functioning, control of protein trafficking between compartments, and processes linked to the suffering and eventual demise of cells (for review see Lukyanenko et al., 2009).

2.5 Mitochondrial involvement in cell apoptosis

Mitochondria are closely involved in the induction of apoptosis. Indeed, the intermembrane space contains several pro-apoptotic proteins which can lead to cell death upon release into the cytosol. Mitochondrial dysfunctions precede and are required for the initiation of the mitochondrial apoptosis pathway (for review see Marzetti et al., 2010). As previously mentioned, subsarcolemmal and intermyofibrillar mitochondria display different susceptibility towards apoptotic stimuli (Adhihetty et al., 2005). Mitochondria may therefore be involved in the pathogenesis of muscle atrophy, in obesity and type 2 diabetes or in response to short-term immobilisation in ageing individuals (Kim et al., 2010; Magne et al., 2011).

3. Transcriptional regulation of mitochondrial oxidative capacity – interaction with fusion-fission dynamics

A number of transcriptional modulators have been implicated in the regulation of muscle mitochondrial biogenesis and OXPHOS activity (figure 3, see also for review Puigserver & Spiegelman, 2003; Chanseaume & Morio, 2009). They include PPAR gamma coactivator 1 alpha (PGC-1α), in cooperation with several factors such as PGC-1β, the peroxisome proliferator-activated receptors (PPAR), the estrogen-related receptor-α (ERRα), the nuclear respiratory factors 1 and 2 (NRF-1 and NRF-2) (Fredenrich & Grimaldi, 2004; Patti et al., 2003; Sparks et al., 2005; Tanaka et al., 2003), or the specificity protein 1 (Sp1), an ubiquitous transcription factor known to regulate the constitutive expression of oxidative OXPHOS genes (Zaid et al., 1999). Sp1 can function as both a positive (e.g. cytochrome c1 and mitochondrial transcription factor A, TFAM) and a negative (e.g. ANT2 and F_1-ATPase beta subunit) regulator of transcription (Yang et al., 2001).

PPARα and PPARβ are involved in the regulation of mitochondrial LCFA oxidative capacity. When bound to their ligands (e.g. LCFA), PPARs form a heterodimeric complex with the retinoid X receptor (RXR) to regulate gene transcription involved in LCFA metabolism. Muscle-specific overexpression of PPARβ in mice was shown to increase oxidative enzyme activities such as citrate synthase or β-hydroxyacyl-CoA dehydrogenase, and to enhance expression of genes implicated in fatty acid catabolism (Luquet et al., 2003).

PGC-1α and PGC-1β, but most importantly PGC-1α, are master modulators of gene expression in skeletal muscle (Moyes, 2003). PGC-1β has been shown to drive the formation of highly oxidative fibers containing type IIX myosin heavy chain (Arany et al., 2007). By contrast, PGC-1α was found to drive the formation of oxidative type I fibres (Lin et al., 2002). In muscle cells, overexpression of PGC-1α was shown to induce the gene expression of NRF-1, NRF-2, TFAM and to activate the expression of genes involved in mitochondrial oxidative capacity (Chabi et al., 2005). PGC-1α gene expression is potently regulated by CREB (cAMP response element-binding protein) binding protein (TORC) 1, a coactivator of CREB (Wu et al., 2006), and by the sirtuin SIRT1 (Amat et al., 2009). Its activity is increased when phosphorylated by p38 stress-activated MAPK (Puigserver et al., 2001) and when deacylated by SIRT1 (Lagouge et al., 2006). Coactivation of ERRα and PPARs by PGC-1α and PGC-1β has been proposed as the major regulatory pathway involved in the control of mitochondrial oxidative capacity (Puigserver & Spiegelman, 2003; Arany et al., 2007; Soriano et al., 2006). For these reasons, alterations in PGC-1α, and to a lesser extent PGC-1β, activity are considered the primary contributors to decreased mitochondrial oxidative capacity in metabolic disorders. Potential intrinsic mechanisms responsible of alterations in mitochondrial biogenesis are reviewed in Chanseaume et al. (2009).

Finally and complementary to mitochondrial biogenesis, recent evidences have demonstrated that the dynamics of mitochondrial network is strongly involved in the control of mitochondrial functioning. It is determined by the balance between fusion and fission events which are govern by mitochondrial proteins such as mitofusin 1 and 2 (Mnf1, Mnf2) and OPA1 for fusion, and dynamin-related protein (DRP1) for fission. Importantly, Mfn2, which gene expression is regulated by PGC-1α and PGC-1β (Pich et al., 2005; Soriano et al., 2006), stimulates respiration, substrate oxidation and OXPHOS subunits expression (Pich et al., 2005). Zorzano et al. (2009) therefore hypothesized that these mitochondrial dynamics proteins play a key role in mitochondrial dysfunction in obesity or in type 2 diabetes and may participate in the development of insulin resistance. This concept is supported by recent studies in muscle (Zorzano et al., 2009) and neurons (Edwards et al., 2010).

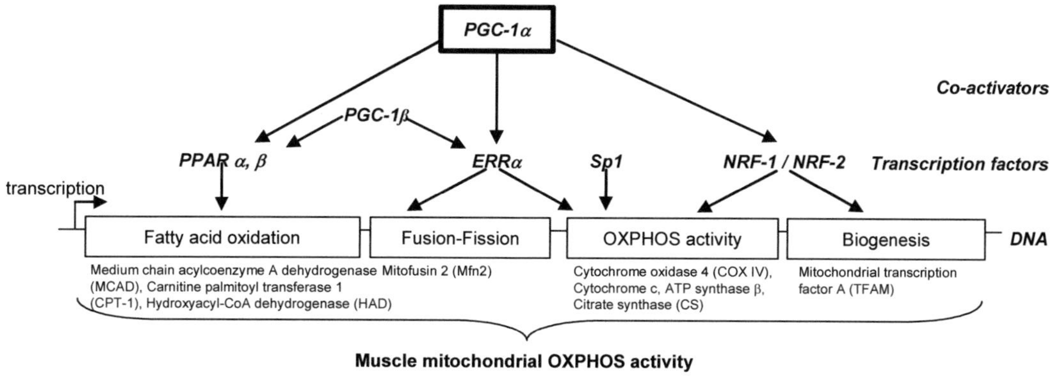

Fig. 3. Major coactivators and transcription factors involved in the regulation of muscle mitochondrial oxidative and phosphorylation (OXPHOS) activity. Non exhaustive key genes, whose expression is regulated by the transcription factors, are given for example.

4. Measurement of muscle mitochondrial OXPHOS activity on muscle biopsy samples

Changes in mitochondrial functioning can be assessed using a battery of biochemical analyses that can often be applied to whole tissue, cells or isolated organelles. These techniques are essential for elucidating intrinsic mechanisms responsible for mitochondrial dysfunctions. However most frequently, they inform about the maximal activity of key enzymes or pathways. In addition, they are limited to the conditions used for the measurements, for example the substrates used to feed the ETC. Therefore, care should be always taken in extrapolating *ex vivo* observations to the *in vivo* situations and generalization should be avoided.

4.1 Samples preparation

Because unfreezing muscle samples brakes mitochondrial structure and alters their functionality, most measurements have to be performed on fresh samples. It is possible to maintain the tissue intact during several hours by using a preservation solution at 4°C until mitochondrial isolation or skinned fiber preparation. Depending on the information required, mitochondrial functioning can be assessed either on isolated organelles or on whole tissue. The latter solution means that one works on tissue homogenates or using the skinned fiber technique. Isolated mitochondria can be obtained by differential centrifugation from at least 80mg of homogenized muscles (Palmer et al., 1977; Capel et al., 2004; supplementary material). This approach is dedicated to the exploration of the organelle intrinsic functioning. Although contaminated by lysosomes, peroxisomes, tubular Golgi membranes, and small amounts of endoplasmic reticulum, the obtained fraction is suitable for respiratory studies (96). Further purification is possible, for example, with Percoll gradients as described by Mickelson et al. (1980) and Graham (2001). Mitochondrial integrity can be monitored by measuring citrate synthase activity before and after freeze-thaw membrane disruption and Triton X-100 addition (Stump et al., 2003). Similarly, mitochondrial purity can be assessed by assessing marker enzymes for lysosomes (β-galactosidase) and peroxisomes (catalase) as discussed by Graham (2001).

By contrast, although evaluated ex-vivo, permeabilized fibers take into account both the intrinsic functioning of mitochondria and the cellular content in mitochondria. Of note, skinned fibers require less muscle sample than the isolation procedure. Fifteen to 20 mg of fresh muscle sample is sufficient for one preparation of saponin-skinned muscle fibers. Briefly as described by Saks et al. (1998), fiber bundles are mechanically separated with tongs and permeabilized with saponin on ice. Bundles are then washed to remove ADP, phosphocreatine, soluble enzymes and metabolites. All steps are critical for obtaining clean skinned fibers for accurately measuring mitochondrial OXPHOS activity and coupling. The time of incubation with saponin depends on the cell type and the animal model. This technique requires therefore a well-trained investigator to assure accurate and repeatable measurements. Novices should follow at the beginning the association between the degree of mechanical separation, time of incubation with saponin and percentage of cells permeabilized and/or respirometric responses. Overpermeabilization should be avoided. The degree of permeabilization can be checked using toluidine blue under optic microscopy. Mitochondrial outer membrane integrity can be also verified during respirometry measurements by checking that addition of cytochrome c had no effect on oxygen consumption.

4.2 Evaluation of mitochondrial density

Mitochondrial density, as well as location, shape and structural integrity, can be reliably assessed using transmission electron microscopy. For that purpose, muscle samples are dissected free of adipose and connective tissue, cut into small pieces (1x1x2mm) and fixed. Transverse sections of 8µm are cut using a cryostat and mounted on slides. Images of 10 random and independent transverse sections of muscle fibers at 36,000 X must be considered. Mitochondrial cross-sectional area (size) and mitochondrial volume density (the fraction of cell volume occupied by mitochondria) are measured by digital imaging morphometry and stereological principles of point sampling, in a blind fashion (Weibel, 1979; Gundersen et al., 1988).

Maximal activity of citrate synthase has been often used as an index of mitochondrial density. This measure is performed on whole tissue homogenates. However, citrate synthase activity can be altered in some physiological situations independently of changes in mitochondrial density. For example, it is well known that aging is associated to a decrease in citrate synthase activity whereas other mitochondrial oxidative enzyme activities are unaltered (Rimbert et al., 2004).

Recently the number of mitochondrial DNA (mtDNA) copy has been considered to reflect mitochondrial content (Wiesner et al., 1992; Barrientos, 2002), the ratio between mtDNA and nuclear DNA has been proposed as a reliable index of mitochondrial density. For that purpose, mitochondrial and nuclear DNAs are extracted during the standard procedure of RNA extraction as described in Chanseaume et al. (2010) and in supplementary material. Purified DNA is ready for quantitative real-time PCR analysis of nuclear and mitochondrial DNA content using primer pairs specific for nuclear (β-actin or myogenin promoter) and mitochondrial (NADH dehydrogenase 1 (ND1), ND2, cytochrome B or cytochrome c oxidase 1 (COX1)) genes (Stump et al., 2003; Petersen et al., 2005; Chanseaume et al., 2010).

4.3 Assessment of maximal activity of key oxidative enzymes

This technique allows the use of frozen samples, either whole tissues, homogenates or isolated organelles. Frozen samples should be kept at -80°C for better preservation of the enzymes integrity. It assesses the maximal activity of the enzyme catalytic site. For that purpose, optimal concentrations in substrates are used to stimulate the enzyme activity. Catalytic activity is determined mostly using spectrophotometry on sample homogenates prepared in sucrose, EDTA Tris-HCl buffer (supplementary material)). For example, complex I activity is assessed measuring NADH oxidation at 340nm. Similarly, complex IV activity is performed at 550nm following the oxidation of reduced cytochrome c. Enzyme activities are often expressed per mg of mitochondrial protein but a most relevant normalisation should be citrate synthase activity or, because of the reason exposed in the previous paragraph, mtDNA content. Methods for measuring the separate activity of all ETC complexes as well as citrate synthase activity are extensively described by Barrientos (2002).

Finally, one can also consider the maximal activity of β-hydroxyacyl-CoA dehydrogenase as a fair index of the beta-oxidation pathway. The assay has been established by Bass et al. (1969). Its principle is based on the disappearance of NADH following reduction of acetoacetyl-CoA to ß-Hydroxybutyryl-CoA (supplementary material).

4.4 Measurement of fatty acid oxidative capacity

Whole muscle LCFA oxidative capacity can be easily determined on fresh muscle homogenates. This technique described by Veerkamp et al. (1983), informs on the maximal ability of muscle tissue to oxidize a specific LCFA. Using two distinct preparations, one can separate peroxisomal from mitochondrial beta-oxidation activities. Of note, our *personnal data* repeatedly showed that the peroxisomal contribution to whole tissue LCFA oxidative capacity averages 10-14%, in humans as well as in rodents.

This technique uses a radiolabelled [1 or U-^{14}C] fatty acid (such as oleate or palmitate for the most commons) bound to albumin at the ratio 4.5:1 (Morio et al., 2001; Rimbert et al., 2004; Tardy et al., 2008). A detailed procedure is provided in supplementary materials. Briefly, total LCFA oxidation is measured using sealed vials containing an aliquot of muscle homogenate in the presence of ATP, NAD+, coenzyme A, L-carnitine, L-malate and cytochrome c. Peroxisomal LCFA oxidation is determined in the presence of mitochondrial oxidation inhibitors (rotenone and antimycin A), but in the absence of L-carnitine and L-malate .

CPT-1 is the key enzyme regulating muscle fatty acid oxidative capacity. It is allosterically inhibited by malonyl-CoA (Rasmussen & Wolfe, 1999). The method measures the amount of palmitoyl-carnitine produced from palmitoyl-CoA and carnitine as described by Kim et al. (2000) and is presented in supplementary materials. CPT-1 activity is measured on freshly isolated mitochondria. It allows assessment of maximal CPT-1 activity as well as its sensitivity to malonyl-CoA inhibition (IC50). Although rarely used, CPT-1 maximal activity can be also assessed from fresh whole muscle homogenates using modification of the above mentioned method (Rimbert et al., 2004). Alternatively, the affinity of mitochondria for palmitoylcarnitine could be assessed using isolated muscle fibers (Ponsot et al., 2005).

4.5 Measurement of mitochondrial respiration

Table 2 summarizes the main substrates used to assess mitochondrial oxidative capacity on isolated organelles or skinned fibers. It also presents the inhibitors required for additional investigation of mitochondrial intrinsic functioning and for measuring state 4 respiration rate. Isolated mitochondria or skinned fiber respiration rates are usually measured at 25°C using an oxygraph system. Higher temperatures, e.g. 30 or 37°C, can be used. This enhances the respiratory rate. Respiration is assayed on 0.25 mg/mL of mitochondrial proteins or 0.5-1.5 mg dried fibers in a specific buffer provided in supplementary materials.

	substrates	inhibitors
TCA cycle	Propionyl-L-carnitine Pyruvate/Palmitoyl-L-carnitine/α-ketoglutarate/L-malate (1mM/5µM/10mM/1mM)	
ß-oxidation	Octanoyl-L-carnitine/L-Malate (100µM/1mM) Palmitoyl-L-carnitine/L-Malate (55µM/1mM)	
Complex I	Glutamate/L-Malate (5mM/2mM) Pyruvate/L-Malate (5mM/2mM) α-ketoglutarate (10mM)	Rotenone (2.4µM) DPI (0.4mM) Amytal (2mM)
Complex II	Succinate* (5mM)	Malonate (10mM) TTFA (1mM)
Complex III	Duroquinol (0.6mM) Glycerol-3Phosphate (5mM)	Antimycin A (10µM) Stigmatellin (6.6 µM)
Complex IV	Ascorbate/TMPD (5mM/1mM)	KCN (0.3mM) Azide (10 mM)
Complex V		Oligomycin B (10µM)
ANT		Atractyloside (60µM) Carboxyatractyloside (250µM) Bongkrekate (1.5µM)
Uncouplers	FCCP (1µM) Valinomycin (3µM)	

Table 2. Substrates, inhibitors and uncouplers used in the polarographic experiments. Concentrations within brackets are indicative. * *used in the presence of rotenone (2 µM); DPI, diphenyliodonium chloride; TTFA, Thenoyltrifluoacetone; TMPD, N,N,N',N'-tetramethyl-p-phenylenediamine; KCN, potassium cyanide; FCCP, carbonyl cyanide p-(trifluoromethoxyl)phenylhydrazone.*

State 2 (non-phosphorylating) respiration is measured in the presence of respiratory substrates without ADP. State 3 (phosphorylated) respiration is measured after the addition of of ADP, saturating concentration leading to maximal ADP-stimulated respiration being 1 mM (Gueguen et al., 2005). A replicate experiment can be done to evaluate uncoupled respiratory rate in the presence of an uncoupler such as carbonylcyanide p-(trifluoromethoxy)phenylhydrazone (FCCP). State 4 respiration is assayed after addition of oligomycin B, an inhibitor of ATP synthase, or after addition of atractyloside, a potent inhibitor of ANT. This measure validates the quality of fiber preparation (notably complete removal of free ADP during washing) if respiration returns to state 2. However, inhibiting ANT may improve the OXPHOS coupling since ANT may be responsible for basal and LCFA-induced uncoupling (Di Paola & Lorusso, 2006). Respiratory control rate is evaluated by dividing state 3 by state 4 rates. Respiration rates are expressed as natom (nat) O/min/µg protein for isolated mitochondria or natom (nat) O/min/mg dried (24 h at 110°C) fibers for skinned fibers.

When differential regulation of respiration by ADP and mitochondrial kinases (creatine kinase, AK2) is of interest, titration protocols with increasing concentration in ADP (from 0.1 to 1 mM) should be performed in the presence or not of 20 mM creatine (creatine kinase activation), or 10 mM glucose (hexokinase activation), 1 mM AMP (AK2 activation), 10 µM Ap5A (AK2 inhibition) (Gueguen et al., 2005). The functional coupling of miCK to energy production could be determined, calculating the affinity for ADP using a combined protocol on permeabilized fibers (N'Guessan et al., 2004).

4.6 Measurement of mitochondrial ATP production

ATP synthase (ATP_{ase}) activity is assayed on freshly isolated mitochondria. Maximal activity is measured spectrophotometrically by monitoring the increase in absorbance at 340 nm using a NADP-linked ADP-regenerating system. Mitochondria are added to the reaction buffer in the presence of glucose, AMP, NADP, ADP, hexokinase, and glucose-6-P dehydrogenase (see supplementary materials) and the reaction is followed at room temperature (Rustin et al., 1994). Similarly, it can also be assessed using a coupled assay between lactate dehydrogenase and pyruvate kinase, NADH reduction being checked at 340 nm (Rustin et al., 1994).

ATP production can be directly measured using bioluminescence kit assay by incubating isolated mitochondria with various substrates of the ETC (Table 2). Blank tubes are used for measuring background and all reactions for a given sample are monitored simultaneously and calibrated with addition of an ATP standard. Mitochondrial ATP production is calculated from the area under the curve (Wibom & Hultman, 1990).

Finally, mitochondrial ATP production can be measured kinetically in parallel with respiration (on isolated mitochondria or permeabilized fibers) as described by Ouhabi et al. (1998). After ADP is added, five 10µl samples are taken every 15 sec in the oxygraph chamber, and frozen in 100µl DMSO before ATP is assayed using a bioluminescence assay kit. ATP production rate is expressed as nmol/min/mg dried fibers. ATP/O is calculated to evaluate coupling of ATP production to ADP-stimulated oxygen consumption (state 3 in nmol O_2/min/mg) (Chanseaume et al., 2010).

4.7 Measurement of mitochondrial ROS production

Using similar incubation conditions than described for respiration or ATP assays, superoxide anion ($O_2^{\bullet -}$) can be assessed on isolated mitochondria using the chemiluminescent probes 2-methyl-6-p methoxyphenylethynylimidazopyazinone (MPEC) (Nakai et al., 2004) or lucigenin (Bis-N-methylacridinium) (Li et al., 1999). Fluorescent sensitive probes such as hydroethidine, especially MitoSOX™ Red which targets the mitochondrial matrix, can also be used. Isolated permeabilized fibers were recently used for $O_2^{\bullet -}$ generation measurement using the triphenylphosphonium Hydroethidine (TTP-HE) reporter (Xu et al., 2010). Signals were analyzed by micellar electrokinetic capillary chromatography coupled to fluorescence detection.

$O_2^{\bullet -}$ rapidly dismutates into H_2O_2 in the presence of mitochondrial SOD which considerably reduce its matrix level. Then the quantification of the more stable H_2O_2 can be assessed using luminol chemiluminescence (Li et al., 1999). H_2O_2 can be also measured using non-fluorescent dyes that become fluorescent upon enzymatic oxidation by H_2O_2 in the presence of horseradish peroxidase. The most commonly used dyes are homovanilic acid (Ruch et al., 1983), 2',7'-dichlorfluorescein-diacetate (DCFH-DA) or Amplex® Red (Chen et al., 2003). Kinetic or global approaches are both adequate for calculating the rate of mitochondrial ROS production. Standard curve is obtained by adding known amounts of H_2O_2 to assay medium in the presence of the reactants. It is critical to quantify background fluorescence, in the absence of mitochondria. Net fluorescence is then calculated minus background and H_2O_2 production is expressed in pmol/mg of protein/min. The heterogeneity of mitochondrial alteration during metabolic disorders could be studied on permeabilized fibers, characterizing the specificity of H_2O_2 production depending on myofiber type (Anderson et al., 2006). If oxygen consumption and ROS production were determined in similar experimental conditions on isolated mitochondria or permeabilized fibers, the free radical leak can be calculated as an indicator of the fraction of electron reducing oxygen to $O_2^{\bullet -}$ (Sanz et al., 2005). It has been shown that this leakage was higher in glycolytic compared to oxidative fibers (Anderson et al., 2006). More recently, new methods were developed to analyze local change in ROS generation on individual isolated fibers. Hence, ROS production could be analyzed by confocal imaging (Shkryl et al., 2009) or real time fluorescence microscopy (Palomero et al., 2008). Although more reliable than $O_2^{\bullet -}$ quantification, the detection of H_2O_2 as an index of $O_2^{\bullet -}$ production has also its limits, i.e., the reaction of $O_2^{\bullet -}$ with other molecules (such as $NO^{\bullet}$), the removal by matrix peroxidase and contamination by H_2O_2 produce within the intermembrane space (see (Murphy, 2009) as a more detailed review on this topic).

4.8 Additional measurement of mitochondrial functionality

Mitochondrial membrane potential can be determined simultaneously with oxygen consumption using the potential-dependent triphenylmethylphosphonium cation ($TPMP^+$) probe as described by Kamo et al. (1979). Development of fluorescent probes sensitive to mitochondrial membrane potential has facilitated the investigation on isolated organelles as well as cells. The most commonly used dyes are rhodamine 123, its derivatives tetramethylrhodamine methyl and ethyl esters (TMRM and TMRE), 3,3'-dihexyloxacarbocyanine,iodide ($DiOC_6(3)$) and 5,5',6,6'-tetrachloro-1,1',3,3'-tetraethyl-benzimidazolcarbocyanine iodide (JC-1). The latter has been proposed as the most reliable probe (Salvioli et al., 1997). Results are usually compared with those obtained in the presence of a mitochondrial uncoupler, such as FCCP, to attain maximum depolarization. Membrane potential could also be determined using isolated permeabilized fibers in a multiwell plate (Xu et al., 2010).

Calcium retention capacity of mitochondria and sensitivity of the permeability transition pore is evaluated on isolated mitochondria using the same incubation buffer and substrates than for respiration, except that 1 µM Calcium Green™-5N is added (Fontaine et al., 1998). Pulses of 10 µM Ca^{2+} are added every minute until pore opening. Specificity of mitochondrial pore opening is assessed by adding cyclosporin A. Comparison between fiber types could be done in a similar approach using permeabilized fibers (Picard et al., 2008).

4.9 Evaluation of mitochondrial biogenesis and fusion-fission dynamics

Supported by steadily increasing literature data, changes in mitochondrial biogenesis and dynamics are relevant mechanisms potentially responsible for mitochondrial dysfunctions. PCR and western blotting analyses are pertinent techniques to investigate these pathways in human samples with limited size (20 to 30 mg). Major proteins potentially involved in these pathways have been described in the previous chapter "Transcriptional regulation of mitochondrial oxidative capacity - interaction with fusion-fission dynamics" and can be targeted using molecular tools.

4.10 Investigation of the mitoproteome

The recent development of genomic tools has considerably improved or knowledge of metabolic disorders within key metabolic tissues. Recently, a proteomic study of mitochondrial proteins (mitoproteome) reported that more than 80% of ETC proteins can be identified (Lefort et al., 2009). The authors were able to reliably detect proteins implicated in ROS generation, scavenging, FA oxidation and apoptosis. One hundred micrograms of human biopsie are required and allow a more than 7 fold enrichment in mitochondrial proteins with a classical isolation procedure as described for respirometry assay. Of note, 30% of identified proteins from the whole tissue proteome are assigned to mitochondria (Yi et al., 2008). Further studies should aim to relate the metabolic disorders and modification of the mitoproteome in insulin sensitive and resistant subjects. This tool combined to transcriptomic analysis should provide key elements to distinguish between mitochondrial functioning defect and mitochondrial density variation during insulin resistance.

5. Conclusions

Exploring mitochondrial functioning in muscle samples, especially from human muscle biopsies, can be achieved using combination of strategies which require a minimal amount of 20mg of tissue for permeabilized fibers for one experimental condition (e.g. respirometry with one substrate), 30mg for molecular exploration and 30mg for an enzyme activity. The most tissue-consuming techniques are those based on isolated mitochondria, which necessitate at least 80mg of tissue for the extraction procedure. Once mitochondrial pellets are obtained, if further purification is not performed, combined and miniaturized methods allow assessing several parameters characterizing mitochondrial functioning (for example respiration, ATP and ROS production and enzyme activities). Hence, 150 to 200mg of tissue sample could be considered as a sufficient condition to build a complete investigation as presented in figure 4. These explorations are however limited in the number of substrates used for testing the ETC.

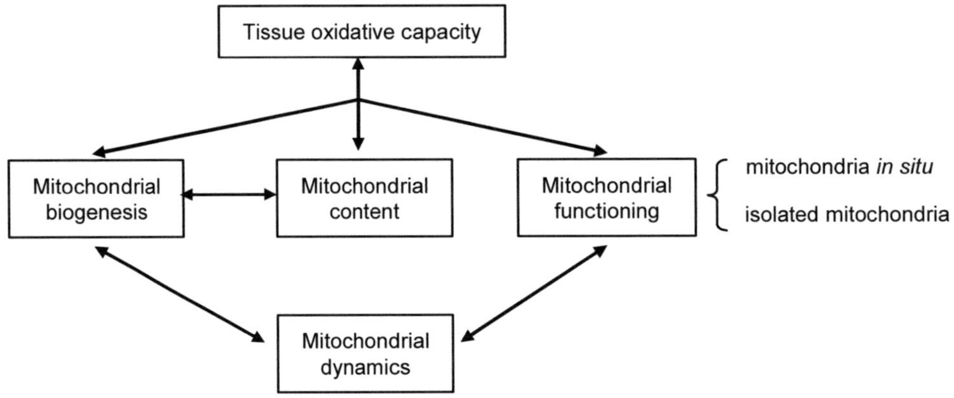

Fig. 4. Main guidelines for exploring mitochondrial functioning in human muscle biopsies.

6. Supplementary materials: buffers composition and protocols

6.1 Preservative solution for isolated fibers

CaK_2EGTA 1.9mM, K_2EGTA 8.1mM, imidazole 20mM, DTT 0.5mM, $MgCl_2$ 9.5mM, MES 53.3mM, taurine 20mM, ATP 2.5mM, phosphocreatine 19mM, pH 7.1.

6.2 Mitochondria isolation buffers and procedure

Tissue grinding: 100mM KCl, 50mM Tris, 5mM MgSO4, 2mM EDTA, 1mM ATP, 0.2% BSA, pH 7.4. To improve the extraction rate of intermyofibrillar mitochondria, treatment with subtilisine type VIII (1.5mg/ml, 5ml/g tissue, incubation 2 to 5 min on ice) is required prior to homogenization.

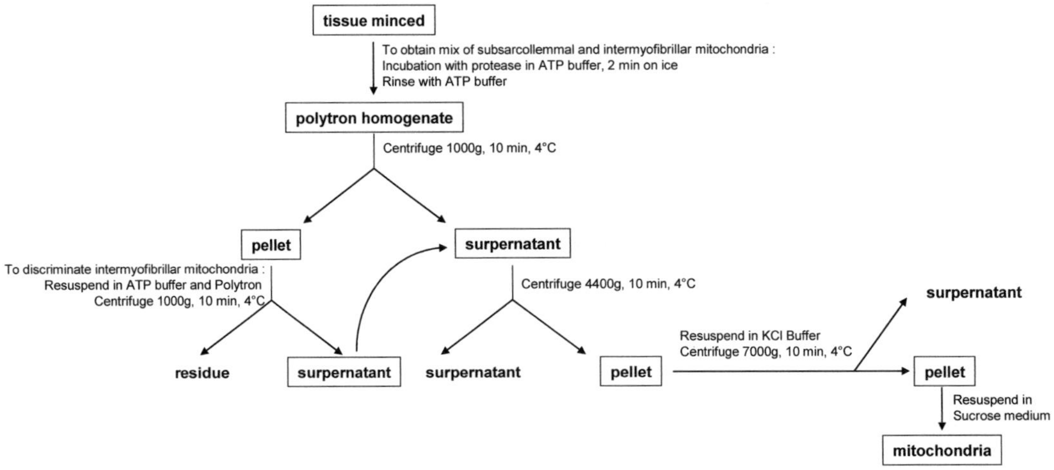

Fig. 5. Procedure for isolating subcellular fractions enriched in mitochondria using differential centrifugation.

KCl buffer: KCl 100mM, Tris 50mM, $MgSO_4$5mM, EDTA 2mM, pH 7.4.

ATP buffer: KCl buffer with ATP 1mM and BSA 0.2%, pH 7.4.

Protease buffer: ATP buffer with subtilisine type VIII (1.5 mg/ml, 5 ml/g tissue).

Sucrose medium: sucrose 0.25M, EGTA 0.1mM, Tris-HCl 10mM, pH 7.4.

6.3 Respiration buffer

CaK_2EGTA 1.9mM, K_2EGTA 8.1mM, imidazole 20mM, DTT 0.5mM, KH_2PO_4 3mM, $MgCl_2$ 4mM, MES 100mM, taurine 20mM, EDTA 20μM and 0.2% BSA.

6.4 Measurement of mitochondrial ATP production

Add freshly isolated mitochondria to the reaction medium containing glucose 400 mM, $MgCl_2$100 mM, KPO_4 100mM, potassium succinate 200mM, AMP 110mM, Hepes 10mM, NADP 7.5mM, ADP 50mM, hexokinase 10μg, and glucose-6-P dehydrogenase 10mg. The total volume in the cuvette is 1 ml. The increase in absorbance at 340nm is followed at room temperature for 3 min (Rustin et al., 1994).

ATP production can also be assessed using a coupled assay between lactate dehydrogenase and pyruvate kinase, NADH reduction being checked at 340 nm. Aliquots of mitochondria (20-40 μg protein) are added to a medium (Tris 50mM, BSA 5mg/ml, $MgCl_2$ 20mM, KCl 50mM, carbonyl cyanide m-chlorophenylhydrazone 15μM, antimycin A 5μM, phosphoenolpyruvate10mM, ATP 2.5mM, 4 units of lactate dehydrogenase and pyruvate kinase, NADH 1mM, pH 8.0) pre-incubated for 5 min at 37°C. The reaction is followed for 3 min before and after oligomycin 3μM is added in order to distinguish the ATPase activity coupled to the ETC (Short et al., 2001).

6.5 DNA purification for mtDNA quantification

Remove the aqueous phase with RNA. Isolate and spun the interphase/organic phase at 12000×g for 5min at 4°C. Remove the remaining aqueous phase to limit contamination with RNA. Add back extraction buffer (4M Guanidine Thiocyanate, 50mM Sodium citrate, 1M Tris; 0.5mL per 1mL of Trizol used for RNA extraction) to each tube and mix for 10 min. Centrifuge at 12000×g for 30min at room temperature. Incubate the upper phase with isopropanol (0.4mL per 1mL of Trizol used for RNA extraction) 5min at room temperature and spun at 12000×g for 15 min at 4°C. Pellets which contain DNA are washed twice with ethanol 70% and spun at 12000×g for 15min at 4°C. Final dissolution is done with sterile water after ethanol removal. DNA concentration is determined spectrophotometrically at 260nm. Total DNA solutions could be stored at -20°C.

6.6 Maximal activity of key oxidative enzymes

Homogeneization buffer for muscle samples: sucrose 0.25mM, EDTA 2mM and Tris-HCl 10mM, pH 7.4.

Buffer for assessing β-hydroxyacyl-CoA dehydrogenase activity: Na_2HPO_4 0.1M, EDTA 2mM, pH 7.5 adjusted with NaH_2PO_4 0.1M, EDTA 2mM. Samples are homogenised in buffer

(Na_2HPO_4 0.1M, EDTA 2mM, pH 7.5 adjusted with NaH_2PO_4 0.1M, EDTA 2mM). 75µl of homogenate is added to 925µl of medium (triethanolamine 100mM, EDTA 5mM, acetoacetyl-CoA 0.1mM, β-NADH 0.45mM, pH 7) and incubated at 30°C during 2 min whilst absorbance is measured at 340nm (Morio et al., 2001).

6.7 Measurement of fatty acid oxidative capacity

At least 50mg of fresh muscle sample is cut into small pieces and crushed in the ice-cold homogeneization buffer (cf 6.6). Total LCFA oxidation is measured using sealed vials in a total volume of 0.5mL containing 75µL of muscle homogenate in a medium (sucrose 25mM, Tris-HCl 75mM, KH_2PO_4 10mM, $MgCl_2$ 5mM, EDTA 1mM, pH 7.4) supplemented with ATP 5mM, NAD^+ 1mM, coenzyme A 0.1mM, L-carnitine 0.5mM, L-malate 0.5mM and cytochrome c 25µM. Peroxisomal LCFA oxidation is determined in the presence of mitochondrial oxidation inhibitors (rotenone and antimycin A) in a medium lacking L-carnitine and L-malate. Blanks are produced by replacing the muscle homogenate with homogeneization buffer.

After 5 min of pre-incubation at 37°C under shaking, the reaction is started by injecting 0.1mL of 600µM of the radiolabelled [^{14}C] fatty acid. Incubation is carried out at 37°C for 30 min and stopped by the addition of 0.2mL of 3M perchloric acid. After 90 min at 4°C, the acid incubation mixture is centrifuged for 5 min at 10,000 g, and the 0.5mL supernatant containing ^{14}C-labelled perchloric acid-soluble products is assayed for radioactivity by liquid scintillation. LCFA oxidation rate is calculated from ^{14}C-labelled perchloric acid-soluble products and expressed in nmoles of fatty acids oxidized per minute per gram wet tissue weight. Mitochondrial oxidation rate is calculated by subtracting the peroxisomal rate from the total oxidation rate. Of note, $^{14}CO_2$ production can be trapped in 0.3mL ethanolamine/ethylene glycol (1:2, v/v) and measured by liquid scintillation.

6.8 Measurement of CPT-1 activity

CPT-1 activity is measured from freshly isolated mitochondria (0.1mg of protein/ml) at 30°C from palmitoyl-L-[methyl-^3H]carnitine formed from L-[methyl-^3H]carnitine (200µM; 10Ci/mol) and palmitoyl-CoA (80µM) in the presence of 1% (w/v) BSA. Increasing concentration of malonyl-CoA (from 0.01 to 600µM) are used for the estimation of the IC50 value (concentration of malonyl-CoA required to achieve 50% inhibition if CPT-1 activity). This method measures the amount of palmitoyl-carnitine produced from palmitoyl-CoA and carnitine and is originately described by Kim et al. (2000).

CPT-1 maximal activity on fresh whole muscle homogenates: 50mg of muscle is homogenized in ice-cold incubation buffer containing KCl 75mM, Hepes 5mM, KCN 2mM, EGTA 0.2mM, DTT 1mM, ATP 5mM, pH 7.3. Fifty microliters of a 5-fold diluted muscle homogenate are preincubated for 5 min at 30°C with 350µl of incubation buffer and 100µl of 80µM palmitoyl-CoA. Reactions are initiated when 50µl of 10mM L-[^3H]carnitine (1µCi) are added at 30°C for 15 min. The reaction is terminated with 1ml of isobutanol. The formed [^3H]palmitoyl-carnitine is extracted with saturated $SO_4(NH_4)_2$ and counted by liquid scintillation. CPT I activity is expressed in nanomoles [^3H]palmitoyl-carnitine per gram of wet tissue per minute corrected for malonyl-CoA (0.3mM)-insensitive [^3H]palmitoyl-carnitine synthesis (Rimbert et al., 2004).

7. References

Abdul-Ghani MA, Jani R, Chavez A, Molina-Carrion M, Tripathy D, Defronzo RA (2009). Mitochondrial reactive oxygen species generation in obese non-diabetic and type 2 diabetic participants. *Diabetologia*; 52(4): 574-582.

Adhihetty PJ, Ljubicic V, Menzies KJ, Hood DA. Differential susceptibility of subsarcolemmal and intermyofibrillar mitochondria to apoptotic stimuli. Am J Physiol Cell Physiol 2005; 289(4): C994-C1001.

Amat R, Planavila A, Chen SL, Iglesias R, Giralt M, Villarroya F (2009). SIRT1 controls the transcription of the peroxisome proliferator-activated receptor-gamma Co-activator-1alpha (PGC-1alpha) gene in skeletal muscle through the PGC-1alpha autoregulatory loop and interaction with MyoD. *J Biol Chem*; 284(33): 21872-21880.

Anderson EJ, Neufer PD (2006). Type II skeletal myofibers possess unique properties that potentiate mitochondrial H(2)O(2) generation. *Am J Physiol Cell Physiol*; 290(3): C844-851.

Arany Z, Lebrasseur N, Morris C, *et al.* (2007). The transcriptional coactivator PGC-1beta drives the formation of oxidative type IIX fibers in skeletal muscle. *Cell Metab*; 5(1): 35-46.

Asmann YW, Stump CS, Short KR, *et al.* (2006). Skeletal muscle mitochondrial functions, mitochondrial DNA copy numbers, and gene transcript profiles in type 2 diabetic and nondiabetic subjects at equal levels of low or high insulin and euglycemia. *Diabetes*; 55(12): 3309-3319.

Bao S, Kennedy A, Wojciechowski B, Wallace P, Ganaway E, Garvey WT (1998). Expression of mRNAs encoding uncoupling proteins in human skeletal muscle: effects of obesity and diabetes. *Diabetes*; 47(12): 1935-1940.

Barja G (1999). Mitochondrial oxygen radical generation and leak: sites of production in states 4 and 3, organ specificity, and relation to aging and longevity. *J Bioenerg Biomembr*; 31(4): 347-366.

Barrientos A. In vivo and in organello assessment of OXPHOS activities. Methods 2002; 26(4): 307-316.

Bass A, Brdiczka D, Eyer P, Hofer S, Pette D (1969). Metabolic differentiation of distinct muscle types at the level of enzymatic organization. *Eur J Biochem*; 10(2): 198-206.

Befroy DE, Petersen KF, Dufour S, *et al.* (2007). Impaired mitochondrial substrate oxidation in muscle of insulin-resistant offspring of type 2 diabetic patients. *Diabetes*; 56(5): 1376-1381.

Benton CR, Nickerson JG, Lally J, *et al.* (2008). Modest PGC-1alpha overexpression in muscle in vivo is sufficient to increase insulin sensitivity and palmitate oxidation in subsarcolemmal, not intermyofibrillar, mitochondria. *J Biol Chem*; 283(7): 4228-4240.

Bezaire V, Seifert EL, Harper ME (2007). Uncoupling protein-3: clues in an ongoing mitochondrial mystery. *FASEB J*; 21(2): 312-324.

Bonnard C, Durand A, Peyrol S, *et al.* (2008). Mitochondrial dysfunction results from oxidative stress in the skeletal muscle of diet-induced insulin-resistant mice. *J Clin Invest*; 118(2): 789-800.

Boushel R, Gnaiger E, Schjerling P, Skovbro M, Kraunsoe R, Dela F (2007). Patients with type 2 diabetes have normal mitochondrial function in skeletal muscle. *Diabetologia*; 50(4): 790-796.

Brons C, Jensen CB, Storgaard H, *et al.* (2008). Mitochondrial function in skeletal muscle is normal and unrelated to insulin action in young men born with low birth weight. *J Clin Endocrinol Metab*; 93(10): 3885-3892.

Capel F, Buffiere C, Patureau Mirand P, Mosoni L (2004). Differential variation of mitochondrial H2O2 release during aging in oxidative and glycolytic muscles in rats. *Mech Ageing Dev*; 125(5): 367-373.

Casteilla L, Rigoulet M, Penicaud L (2001). Mitochondrial ROS metabolism: modulation by uncoupling proteins. *IUBMB Life*; 52(3-5): 181-188.

Chabi B, Adhihetty PJ, Ljubicic V, Hood DA (2005). How is mitochondrial biogenesis affected in mitochondrial disease? *Med Sci Sports Exerc*; 37(12): 2102-2110.

Chanseaume E, Morio B (2009). Potential mechanisms of muscle mitochondrial dysfunction in aging and obesity and cellular consequences. *Int J Mol Sci*; 10(1): 306-324.

Chanseaume E, Barquissau V, Salles J, *et al.* (2010). Muscle mitochondrial oxidative phosphorylation activity, but not content, is altered with abdominal obesity in sedentary men: synergism with changes in insulin sensitivity. *J Clin Endocrinol Metab*; 95(6): 2948-2956.

Chavez JA, Holland WL, Bar J, Sandhoff K, Summers SA (2005). Acid ceramidase overexpression prevents the inhibitory effects of saturated fatty acids on insulin signaling. *J Biol Chem*; 280(20): 20148-20153.

Chen Q, Vazquez EJ, Moghaddas S, Hoppel CL, Lesnefsky EJ (2003). Production of reactive oxygen species by mitochondria: central role of complex III. *J Biol Chem*; 278(38): 36027-36031.

Coll T, Jove M, Rodriguez-Calvo R, *et al.* (2006). Palmitate-mediated downregulation of peroxisome proliferator-activated receptor-gamma coactivator 1alpha in skeletal muscle cells involves MEK1/2 and nuclear factor-kappaB activation. *Diabetes*; 55(10): 2779-2787.

Debard C, Laville M, Berbe V, *et al.* (2004). Expression of key genes of fatty acid oxidation, including adiponectin receptors, in skeletal muscle of Type 2 diabetic patients. *Diabetologia*; 47(5): 917-925.

Deluca HF, Engstrom GW (1961). Calcium uptake by rat kidney mitochondria. *Proc Natl Acad Sci U S A*; 47: 1744-1750.

Di Paola M, Lorusso M (2006). Interaction of free fatty acids with mitochondria: coupling, uncoupling and permeability transition. *Biochim Biophys Acta;* 1757(9-10): 1330-7.

Edwards JL, Quattrini A, Lentz SI, *et al.* (2010). Diabetes regulates mitochondrial biogenesis and fission in mouse neurons. *Diabetologia*; 53(1): 160-169.

Fontaine E, Eriksson O, Ichas F, Bernardi P (1998). Regulation of the permeability transition pore in skeletal muscle mitochondria. Modulation By electron flow through the respiratory chain complex I. *J Biol Chem*; 273(20): 12662-12668.

Fredenrich A, Grimaldi PA (2004). Roles of peroxisome proliferator-activated receptor delta in skeletal muscle function and adaptation. *Curr Opin Clin Nutr Metab Care*; 7(4): 377-381.

Garcia-Martinez C, Marotta M, Moore-Carrasco R, *et al.* (2005). Impact on fatty acid metabolism and differential localization of FATP1 and FAT/CD36 proteins delivered in cultured human muscle cells. *Am J Physiol Cell Physiol*; 288(6): C1264-1272.

Graham JM (2001). Purification of a crude mitochondrial fraction by density-gradient centrifugation. *Curr Protoc Cell Biol*; Chapter 3: Unit 3 4.

Gueguen N, Lefaucheur L, Ecolan P, Fillaut M, Herpin P (2005). Ca2+-activated myosin-ATPases, creatine and adenylate kinases regulate mitochondrial function according to myofibre type in rabbit. *J Physiol*; 564(Pt 3): 723-735.

Gundersen HJ, Bendtsen TF, Korbo L, *et al.* (1988). Some new, simple and efficient stereological methods and their use in pathological research and diagnosis. *APMIS*; 96(5): 379-394.

Gunter KK, Gunter TE (1994). Transport of calcium by mitochondria. *J Bioenerg Biomembr*; 26(5): 471-485.

Hand SC, Menze MA (2008). Mitochondria in energy-limited states: mechanisms that blunt the signaling of cell death. *J Exp Biol*; 211(Pt 12): 1829-1840.

He J, Watkins S, Kelley DE (2001). Skeletal muscle lipid content and oxidative enzyme activity in relation to muscle fiber type in type 2 diabetes and obesity. *Diabetes*; 50(4): 817-823.

Hegarty BD, Furler SM, Ye J, Cooney GJ, Kraegen EW (2003). The role of intramuscular lipid in insulin resistance. *Acta Physiol Scand*; 178(4): 373-383.

Heilbronn LK, Gan SK, Turner N, Campbell LV, Chisholm DJ (2007). Markers of mitochondrial biogenesis and metabolism are lower in overweight and obese insulin-resistant subjects. *J Clin Endocrinol Metab*; 92(4): 1467-1473.

Holloway GP, Thrush AB, Heigenhauser GJ, *et al.* (2007). Skeletal muscle mitochondrial FAT/CD36 content and palmitate oxidation are not decreased in obese women. *Am J Physiol Endocrinol Metab*; 292(6): E1782-1789.

Hoppe UC (2010). Mitochondrial calcium channels. *FEBS Lett*; 584(10): 1975-1981.

Howald H, Hoppeler H, Claassen H, Mathieu O, Straub R (1985). Influences of endurance training on the ultrastructural composition of the different muscle fiber types in humans. *Pflugers Arch*; 403(4): 369-376.

Jouaville LS, Pinton P, Bastianutto C, Rutter GA, Rizzuto R (1999). Regulation of mitochondrial ATP synthesis by calcium: evidence for a long-term metabolic priming. *Proc Natl Acad Sci U S A*; 96(24): 13807-13812.

Kamo N, Muratsugu M, Hongoh R, Kobatake Y (1979). Membrane potential of mitochondria measured with an electrode sensitive to tetraphenyl phosphonium and relationship between proton electrochemical potential and phosphorylation potential in steady state. *J Membr Biol*; 49(2): 105-121.

Kelley DE, He J, Menshikova EV, Ritov VB (2002). Dysfunction of mitochondria in human skeletal muscle in type 2 diabetes. *Diabetes*; 51(10): 2944-2950.

Kewalramani G, Bilan PJ, Klip A (2010). Muscle insulin resistance: assault by lipids, cytokines and local macrophages. *Curr Opin Clin Nutr Metab Care*; 13(4): 382-390.

Kim JY, Hickner RC, Cortright RL, Dohm GL, Houmard JA (2000). Lipid oxidation is reduced in obese human skeletal muscle. *Am J Physiol Endocrinol Metab*; 279(5): E1039-1044.

Kim TN, Park MS, Yang SJ, *et al.* (2010). Prevalence and determinant factors of sarcopenia in patients with type 2 diabetes: the Korean Sarcopenic Obesity Study (KSOS). *Diabetes Care*; 33(7): 1497-1499.

Korshunov SS, Skulachev VP, Starkov AA (1997). High protonic potential actuates a mechanism of production of reactive oxygen species in mitochondria. *FEBS Lett*; 416(1): 15-18.

Koves TR, Noland RC, Bates AL, Henes ST, Muoio DM, Cortright RN (2005). Subsarcolemmal and intermyofibrillar mitochondria play distinct roles in regulating skeletal muscle fatty acid metabolism. *Am J Physiol Cell Physiol*; 288(5): C1074-1082.

Krook A, Digby J, O'Rahilly S, Zierath JR, Wallberg-Henriksson H (1998). Uncoupling protein 3 is reduced in skeletal muscle of NIDDM patients. *Diabetes*; 47(9): 1528-1531.

Lagouge M, Argmann C, Gerhart-Hines Z, *et al.* (2006). Resveratrol improves mitochondrial function and protects against metabolic disease by activating SIRT1 and PGC-1alpha. *Cell*; 127(6): 1109-1122.

Lefort N, Yi Z, Bowen B, *et al.* (2009). Proteome profile of functional mitochondria from human skeletal muscle using one-dimensional gel electrophoresis and HPLC-ESI-MS/MS. *J Proteomics*; 72(6): 1046-1060.

Leloup C, Casteilla L, Carrière A, Galinier A, Benani A, Carneiro L, Pénicaud L (2011). Balancing mitochondrial redox signaling: a key point in metabolic regulation. *Antioxid Redox Signal*; 14(3):519-30.

Li B, Nolte LA, Ju JS, *et al.* (2000). Skeletal muscle respiratory uncoupling prevents diet-induced obesity and insulin resistance in mice. *Nat Med*; 6(10): 1115-1120.

Li Y, Zhu H, Trush MA (1999). Detection of mitochondria-derived reactive oxygen species production by the chemilumigenic probes lucigenin and luminol. *Biochim Biophys Acta*; 1428(1): 1-12.

Lin J, Wu H, Tarr PT, *et al.* (2002). Transcriptional co-activator PGC-1 alpha drives the formation of slow-twitch muscle fibres. *Nature*; 418(6899): 797-801.

Liu Y, Fiskum G, Schubert D (2002). Generation of reactive oxygen species by the mitochondrial electron transport chain. *J Neurochem*; 80(5): 780-787.

Lukyanenko V, Chikando A, Lederer WJ (2009). Mitochondria in cardiomyocyte Ca2+ signaling. *Int J Biochem Cell Biol*; 41(10): 1957-1971.

Luquet S, Lopez-Soriano J, Holst D, *et al.* (2003). Peroxisome proliferator-activated receptor delta controls muscle development and oxidative capability. *FASEB J*; 17(15): 2299-2301.

Magne H, Savary-Auzeloux I, Vazeille E, Claustre A, Attaix D, Anne L, Véronique SL, Philippe G, Dardevet D, Combaret L (2011). Lack of muscle recovery after immobilization in old rats does not result from a defect in normalization of the ubiquitin-proteasome and the caspase-dependent apoptotic pathways. *J Physiol*; 589(Pt 3):511-24..

Marzetti E, Hwang JC, Lees HA, *et al.* (2010). Mitochondrial death effectors: relevance to sarcopenia and disuse muscle atrophy. *Biochim Biophys Acta*; 1800(3): 235-244.

McCormack JG, Halestrap AP, Denton RM (1990). Role of calcium ions in regulation of mammalian intramitochondrial metabolism. *Physiol Rev*; 70(2): 391-425.

McGarry JD, Brown NF (1997). The mitochondrial carnitine palmitoyltransferase system. From concept to molecular analysis. *Eur J Biochem*; 244(1): 1-14.

Mickelson JR, Greaser ML, Marsh BB (1980). Purification of skeletal-muscle mitochondria by density-gradient centrifugation with Percoll. *Anal Biochem*; 109(2): 255-260.

Mitchell P (1961). Coupling of phosphorylation to electron and hydrogen transfer by a chemi-osmotic type of mechanism. *Nature*; 191: 144-148.

Miwa S, Brand MD (2003). Mitochondrial matrix reactive oxygen species production is very sensitive to mild uncoupling. *Biochem Soc Trans*; 31(Pt 6): 1300-1301.

Mollica MP, Lionetti L, Crescenzo R, *et al.* (2006). Heterogeneous bioenergetic behaviour of subsarcolemmal and intermyofibrillar mitochondria in fed and fasted rats. *Cell Mol Life Sci*; 63(3): 358-366.

Montuschi P, Barnes PJ, Roberts LJ 2nd (2004). Isoprostanes: markers and mediators of oxidative stress. *FASEB J*; 18(15): 1791-1800.

Mootha VK, Lindgren CM, Eriksson KF, *et al.* (2003). PGC-1alpha-responsive genes involved in oxidative phosphorylation are coordinately downregulated in human diabetes. *Nat Genet*; 34(3): 267-273.

Morino K, Petersen KF, Dufour S, *et al.* (2005). Reduced mitochondrial density and increased IRS-1 serine phosphorylation in muscle of insulin-resistant offspring of type 2 diabetic parents. *J Clin Invest*; 115(12): 3587-3593.

Morio B, Hocquette JF, Montaurier C, *et al.* (2001). Muscle fatty acid oxidative capacity is a determinant of whole body fat oxidation in elderly people. *Am J Physiol Endocrinol Metab*; 280(1): E143-149.

Moser MD, Matsuzaki S, Humphries KM (2009). Inhibition of succinate-linked respiration and complex II activity by hydrogen peroxide. *Arch Biochem Biophys*; 488(1): 69-75.

Moyes CD (2003). Controlling muscle mitochondrial content. *J Exp Biol*; 206(Pt 24): 4385-4391.

Murphy MP (2009). How mitochondria produce reactive oxygen species. *Biochem J*; 417(1): 1-13.

Nair KS, Bigelow ML, Asmann YW, *et al.* (2008). Asian Indians have enhanced skeletal muscle mitochondrial capacity to produce ATP in association with severe insulin resistance. *Diabetes*; 57(5): 1166-1175.

Nakai D, Shimizu T, Nojiri H, *et al.* coq7/clk-1 regulates mitochondrial respiration and the generation of reactive oxygen species via coenzyme Q. Aging Cell 2004; 3(5): 273-281.

N'Guessan B, Zoll J, Ribera F, *et al.* (2004). Evaluation of quantitative and qualitative aspects of mitochondrial function in human skeletal and cardiac muscles. *Mol Cell Biochem*; 256-257(1-2): 267-280.

Nicholls DG, Chalmers S (2004). The integration of mitochondrial calcium transport and storage. *J Bioenerg Biomembr*; 36(4): 277-281.

Nulton-Persson AC, Szweda LI (2001). Modulation of mitochondrial function by hydrogen peroxide. *J Biol Chem*; 276(26): 23357-23361.

Ortenblad N, Mogensen M, Petersen I, *et al.* (2005). Reduced insulin-mediated citrate synthase activity in cultured skeletal muscle cells from patients with type 2 diabetes: evidence for an intrinsic oxidative enzyme defect. *Biochim Biophys Acta*; 1741(1-2): 206-214.

Ouhabi R, Boue-Grabot M, Mazat JP (1998). Mitochondrial ATP synthesis in permeabilized cells: assessment of the ATP/O values in situ. *Anal Biochem*; 263(2): 169-175.

Palmer JW, Tandler B, Hoppel CL (1977). Biochemical properties of subsarcolemmal and interfibrillar mitochondria isolated from rat cardiac muscle. *J Biol Chem*; 252(23): 8731-8739.

Palomero J, Pye D, Kabayo T, Spiller DG, Jackson MJ (2008). In situ detection and measurement of intracellular reactive oxygen species in single isolated mature skeletal muscle fibers by real time fluorescence microscopy. *Antioxid Redox Signal*; 10(8): 1463-1474.

Patti ME, Butte AJ, Crunkhorn S, *et al.* (2003)Coordinated reduction of genes of oxidative metabolism in humans with insulin resistance and diabetes: Potential role of PGC1 and NRF1. *Proc Natl Acad Sci U S A*; 100(14): 8466-8471.

Petersen KF, Dufour S, Befroy D, Garcia R, Shulman GI (2004). Impaired mitochondrial activity in the insulin-resistant offspring of patients with type 2 diabetes. *N Engl J Med*; 350(7): 664-671.

Petersen KF, Dufour S, Shulman GI (2005). Decreased insulin-stimulated ATP synthesis and phosphate transport in muscle of insulin-resistant offspring of type 2 diabetic parents. *PLoS Med*; 2(9): e233.

Petersen KF, Shulman GI (2006). Etiology of insulin resistance. *Am J Med*; 119(5 Suppl 1): S10-16.

Picard M, Csukly K, Robillard ME, *et al.* (2008). Resistance to Ca2+-induced opening of the permeability transition pore differs in mitochondria from glycolytic and oxidative muscles. *Am J Physiol Regul Integr Comp Physiol*; 295(2): R659-668.

Pich S, Bach D, Briones P, *et al.* (2005). The Charcot-Marie-Tooth type 2A gene product, Mfn2, up-regulates fuel oxidation through expression of OXPHOS system. *Hum Mol Genet*; 14(11): 1405-1415.

Ponsot E, Zoll J, N'Guessan B, *et al.* (2005). Mitochondrial tissue specificity of substrates utilization in rat cardiac and skeletal muscles. *J Cell Physiol*; 203(3): 479-486.

Puigserver P, Rhee J, Lin J, *et al.* (2001). Cytokine stimulation of energy expenditure through p38 MAP kinase activation of PPARgamma coactivator-1. *Mol Cell*; 8(5): 971-982.

Puigserver P, Spiegelman BM (2003). Peroxisome proliferator-activated receptor-gamma coactivator 1 alpha (PGC-1 alpha): transcriptional coactivator and metabolic regulator. *Endocr Rev*; 24(1): 78-90.

Rasmussen BB, Wolfe RR (1999). Regulation of fatty acid oxidation in skeletal muscle. *Annu Rev Nutr*; 19: 463-484.

Rimbert V, Boirie Y, Bedu M, Hocquette JF, Ritz P, Morio B (2004). Muscle fat oxidative capacity is not impaired by age but by physical inactivity: association with insulin sensitivity. *FASEB J*; 18(6): 737-739.

Rimbert V, Vidal H, Duche P, *et al.* (2009). Rapid down-regulation of mitochondrial fat metabolism in human muscle after training cessation is dissociated from changes in insulin sensitivity. *FEBS Lett*; 583(17): 2927-2933.

Ritov VB, Menshikova EV, He J, Ferrell RE, Goodpaster BH, Kelley DE (2005). Deficiency of subsarcolemmal mitochondria in obesity and type 2 diabetes. *Diabetes*; 54(1): 8-14.

Ritov VB, Menshikova EV, Azuma K, *et al.* (2010). Deficiency of electron transport chain in human skeletal muscle mitochondria in type 2 diabetes mellitus and obesity. *Am J Physiol Endocrinol Metab*; 298(1): E49-58.

Rizzuto R, Pinton P, Carrington W, *et al.* (1998). Close contacts with the endoplasmic reticulum as determinants of mitochondrial Ca2+ responses. Science 1998; 280(5370): 1763-1766.

Ruch W, Cooper PH, Baggiolini M. Assay of H2O2 production by macrophages and neutrophils with homovanillic acid and horse-radish peroxidase. *J Immunol Methods*; 63(3): 347-357.

Rustin P, Chretien D, Bourgeron T, *et al.* (1994). Biochemical and molecular investigations in respiratory chain deficiencies. *Clin Chim Acta*; 228(1): 35-51.

Saks VA, Khuchua ZA, Vasilyeva EV, Belikova O, Kuznetsov AV (1994). Metabolic compartmentation and substrate channelling in muscle cells. Role of coupled creatine kinases in in vivo regulation of cellular respiration--a synthesis. *Mol Cell Biochem*; 133-134: 155-192.

Saks VA, Veksler VI, Kuznetsov AV, *et al.* (1998). Permeabilized cell and skinned fiber techniques in studies of mitochondrial function in vivo. *Mol Cell Biochem*; 184(1-2): 81-100.

Salvioli S, Ardizzoni A, Franceschi C, Cossarizza A (1997). JC-1, but not DiOC6(3) or rhodamine 123, is a reliable fluorescent probe to assess delta psi changes in intact cells: implications for studies on mitochondrial functionality during apoptosis. *FEBS Lett*; 411(1): 77-82.

Samec S, Seydoux J, Dulloo AG (1999). Post-starvation gene expression of skeletal muscle uncoupling protein 2 and uncoupling protein 3 in response to dietary fat levels and fatty acid composition: a link with insulin resistance. *Diabetes*; 48(2): 436-441.

Sanz A, Caro P, Ibanez J, Gomez J, Gredilla R, Barja G (2005). Dietary restriction at old age lowers mitochondrial oxygen radical production and leak at complex I and oxidative DNA damage in rat brain. *J Bioenerg Biomembr*; 37(2): 83-90.

Schrauwen P, Hesselink M (2002). UCP2 and UCP3 in muscle controlling body metabolism. *J Exp Biol*; 205(Pt 15): 2275-2285.

Schrauwen-Hinderling VB, Kooi ME, Hesselink MK, *et al.* (2007). Impaired in vivo mitochondrial function but similar intramyocellular lipid content in patients with type 2 diabetes mellitus and BMI-matched control subjects. *Diabetologia*; 50(1): 113-120.

Seifert EL, Estey C, Xuan JY, Harper ME (2010). Electron transport chain-dependent and -independent mechanisms of mitochondrial H2O2 emission during long-chain fatty acid oxidation. *J Biol Chem*; 285(8): 5748-5758.

Shkryl VM, Martins AS, Ullrich ND, Nowycky MC, Niggli E, Shirokova N (2009). Reciprocal amplification of ROS and Ca(2+) signals in stressed mdx dystrophic skeletal muscle fibers. *Pflugers Arch*; 458(5): 915-928.

Short KR, Nygren J, barazzoni R, Levine J, Nair KS (2001). T(3) increases mitochondrial ATP production in oxidative muscle despite increased expression of UCP2 and -3. *Am J Physiol Endocr Metab*; 285(5):E761-769.

Shulman GI (2000). Cellular mechanisms of insulin resistance. *J Clin Invest*; 106(2): 171-176.

Skulachev VP (1997). Membrane-linked systems preventing superoxide formation. *Biosci Rep*; 17(3): 347-366.

Slawik M, Vidal-Puig AJ (2006). Lipotoxicity, overnutrition and energy metabolism in aging. *Ageing Res Rev*; 5(2): 144-164.

Soriano FX, Liesa M, Bach D, Chan DC, Palacin M, Zorzano A (2006). Evidence for a mitochondrial regulatory pathway defined by peroxisome proliferator-activated receptor-gamma coactivator-1 alpha, estrogen-related receptor-alpha, and mitofusin 2. *Diabetes*; 55(6): 1783-1791.

Sparks LM, Xie H, Koza RA, *et al.* (2005). A high-fat diet coordinately downregulates genes required for mitochondrial oxidative phosphorylation in skeletal muscle. *Diabetes*; 54(7): 1926-1933.

Stump CS, Short KR, Bigelow ML, Schimke JM, Nair KS (2003). Effect of insulin on human skeletal muscle mitochondrial ATP production, protein synthesis, and mRNA transcripts. *Proc Natl Acad Sci U S A*; 100(13): 7996-8001.

Szendroedi J, Schmid AI, Chmelik M, *et al.* (2007). Muscle mitochondrial ATP synthesis and glucose transport/phosphorylation in type 2 diabetes. *PLoS Med*; 4(5): e154.

Tanaka T, Yamamoto J, Iwasaki S, *et al.* (2003). Activation of peroxisome proliferator-activated receptor delta induces fatty acid beta-oxidation in skeletal muscle and attenuates metabolic syndrome. *Proc Natl Acad Sci U S A*; 100(26): 15924-15929.

Tardy AL, Giraudet C, Rousset P, *et al.* (2008). Effects of trans MUFA from dairy and industrial sources on muscle mitochondrial function and insulin sensitivity. *J Lipid Res*; 49(7): 1445-1455.

Territo PR, Mootha VK, French SA, Balaban RS (2000). Ca(2+) activation of heart mitochondrial oxidative phosphorylation: role of the F(0)/F(1)-ATPase. *Am J Physiol Cell Physiol*; 278(2): C423-435.

Toledo FG, Menshikova EV, Azuma K, *et al.* (2008). Mitochondrial capacity in skeletal muscle is not stimulated by weight loss despite increases in insulin action and decreases in intramyocellular lipid content. *Diabetes*; 57(4): 987-994.

Vasington FD, Murphy JV (1962). Ca ion uptake by rat kidney mitochondria and its dependence on respiration and phosphorylation. *J Biol Chem*; 237: 2670-2677.

Veerkamp JH, Van Moerkerk HT, Glatz JF, Van Hinsbergh VW (1983). Incomplete palmitate oxidation in cell-free systems of rat and human muscles. *Biochim Biophys Acta*; 753(3): 399-410.

Votyakova TV, Reynolds IJ (2001). DeltaPsi(m)-Dependent and -independent production of reactive oxygen species by rat brain mitochondria. *J Neurochem*; 79(2): 266-277.

Weibel ER (1979). Practical Methods for Biological Morphometry. *Stereological Methods*, New York, Academic Press; Volumes 1 and 2.

Wibom R, Hultman E (1990). ATP production rate in mitochondria isolated from microsamples of human muscle. *Am J Physiol*; 259(2 Pt 1): E204-209.

Wiesner RJ, Ruegg JC, Morano I (1992). Counting target molecules by exponential polymerase chain reaction: copy number of mitochondrial DNA in rat tissues. *Biochem Biophys Res Commun*; 183(2): 553-559.

Wilson DF, Owen CS, Holian A (1977). Control of mitochondrial respiration: a quantitative evaluation of the roles of cytochrome c and oxygen. *Arch Biochem Biophys*; 182(2): 749-762.

Wu Z, Huang X, Feng Y, *et al.* (2006). Transducer of regulated CREB-binding proteins (TORCs) induce PGC-1alpha transcription and mitochondrial biogenesis in muscle cells. *Proc Natl Acad Sci U S A*; 103(39): 14379-14384.

Xu X, Thompson LV, Navratil M, Arriaga EA (2010). Analysis of superoxide production in single skeletal muscle fibers. *Anal Chem*; 82(11): 4570-4576.

Yang X, Su K, Roos MD, Chang Q, Paterson AJ, Kudlow JE (2001). O-linkage of N-acetylglucosamine to Sp1 activation domain inhibits its transcriptional capability. *Proc Natl Acad Sci U S A*; 98(12): 6611-6616.

Yi Z, Bowen BP, Hwang H, *et al.* (2008). Global relationship between the proteome and transcriptome of human skeletal muscle. *J Proteome Res*; 7(8): 3230-3241.

Zaid A, Li R, Luciakova K, Barath P, Nery S, Nelson BD (1999). On the role of the general transcription factor Sp1 in the activation and repression of diverse mammalian oxidative phosphorylation genes. *J Bioenerg Biomembr*; 31(2): 129-135.

Zoll J, Koulmann N, Bahi L, Ventura-Clapier R, Bigard AX (2003). Quantitative and qualitative adaptation of skeletal muscle mitochondria to increased physical activity. *J Cell Physiol*; 194(2): 186-193.

Zorzano A, Liesa M, Palacin M (2009). Role of mitochondrial dynamics proteins in the pathophysiology of obesity and type 2 diabetes. *Int J Biochem Cell Biol*; 41(10): 1846-1854.

6

Metabolic Exploration of Muscle Biopsy

A.L. Charles, S. Dufour, T.N. Tran, J. Bouitbir, B. Geny and J. Zoll
University of Strasbourg, EA 3072, Medicine Faculty
France

1. Introduction

It has been well established that in several chronic diseases such as in chronic obstructive pulmonary disease (COPD), diabetes, cancer or congestive heart failure patients, next to central dysfunctions, the patients develop some systemic consequences that can lead to peripheral muscle dysfunction. Some important clinical implications such as reduced exercise capacity, reduced quality of life and lower survival in these patients are related to changes in muscle structure (mass) and function (power and endurance) (Maltais et al., 1996; 1999; Mettauer et al., 2006). In chronic disease, peripheral perturbations generally include neurohormonal and inflammatory changes, microvascular dysfunction, endothelial abnormalities, tissue wasting, apoptosis and energetic imbalance in skeletal muscle cells, causing reduced exercise capacity. These multisystem abnormalities contribute to the progressive worsening of the disease, and ultimately, lead to premature death. Among the numerous skeletal muscle cell changes that occur in chronic disease, energetic dysfunction has received renewed attention in the last decade and is increasingly considered to be a possible unifying mechanism in the development of muscle failure (Mettauer et al., 2006).

The mitochondrial impairments seem to be central in the development of energy dysfunction. Indeed, morphometric analysis of vastus lateralis from chronic heart failure patients revealed a decreased volume density of the mitochondria and decreased surface of the cristae in proportion with the decrease in VO2peak (Drexler, 1992). The percentage of the mitochondria stained for cytochrome oxidase (COX) is also reduced but improves with training (Hambrecht et al., 1995). Muscle enzymatic analysis as citrate synthase activity was decreased (De Sousa et al., 2000; Mettauer et al., 2001; Williams et al., 2004). Mitochondrial dysfunction has also been implicated in the pathology of chronic metabolic disease characterized by insulin resistance such as obesity, type 2 diabetes mellitus, and aging (Johannsen & Ravussin, 2009). In some chronic diseases as heart failure, skeletal muscle abnormalities resemble those induced by physical deconditioning, but some features argue for a generalized metabolic myopathy.

These observations shown in several studies were obtained using various experimental techniques such as nuclear magnetic resonance (NMR) spectroscopy, measurement of mitochondrial function in situ or in vitro by oxygraphy, proteomics and genomics in human or animal models, which have all revealed muscular energetic perturbations. Indeed, mitochondria play a central role in hereditary mitochondrial diseases, ischemia reperfusion injury, heart failure, metabolic syndrome, neurodegenerative diseases and cancer. Thus, comprehension of mitochondrial function regulation is fundamental in order to enlarge the knowledge in the field of mitochondrial physiology, and above all in order to better diagnose the implication of mitochondria in many diseases. Direct assessment of mitochondrial function by measuring coupled respiration and ATP synthesis provides more full information, and the study of oxidative phosphorylation in skeletal muscles is an important initial screening procedure for the potential presence of mitochondrial diseases. At the fundamental level, comprehension of the mechanisms governing mitochondrial function as well as mitochondrial biogenesis remain to be explored in details with more and more molecular and cellular approaches.

2. Different types of skeletal muscle are available

2.1 Different muscle types

In function of pathologies, clinical symptoms, experimental conditions or physical exercise type, the choice of skeletal muscle could be different. Deltoid and Vastus Lateralis muscles are the skeletal muscles classically explored. But muscular biopsy could also be carried out in Tibialis anterior and Gastrocnemius muscles. During chirurgical intervention, some other striated muscles such as pectoral, respiratory or backbone muscles could also be explored. For that, researchers need to obtain the informed consent from all patients and the study has to be approved by the institutional ethical review board.

2.2 Different muscle fibres

In function of muscle types, the composition and the properties of muscle fibres will be different. Indeed, an abundance of literature shows that human skeletal muscles are made of a mixed nature, depending on its function. Muscles are composed of various proportions of the three fibre types I, IIa and IIx (or IIb depending on the species), each having specific contractile and metabolic characteristics. Fibre type composition exhibits great plasticity that depends on activity, mechanical load, hormonal status and age (Baldwin et al., 1975; Schiaffino & Reggiani, 1996; Fluck & Hoppeler, 2003). Moreover, quantitative differences between muscles in terms of mitochondrial and capillary density, enzymatic profile and content of high-energy phosphates have been widely reported (Table 1, figure1).

	Skeletal muscle fibres			**Cardiac fibres**
fibers type	Slow-oxidative	Fast-oxidative	Fast-glycolytic	
	Type I	Type IIa	Type IIx, Type IIb	
Myosin ATPase activity	Low	High	High	Low
Speed of contraction	Slow	Fast	Fast	Slow
Resistance to fatigue	High	Intermediate	Low	Very high
Oxidative capacity	High	High	Low	Very high
Mitochondria density	High	High	Low	Very high
Myoglobin content	High	High	Low	Very high
Glycogen content	Low	Intermediate	High	Very low
Citrate synthase	High activity	High activity	Low activity	Very high activity
miCK	High activity	High activity	Low activity	Very high activity

Table 1. The different characteristics of muscle fibres. For the sake of simplicity fibre types have been separated in slow oxidative type I, fast oxidative type IIa and fast glycolytic type IIb. miCK: mitochondrial isoenzyme of creatine kinase. (Mettauer et al., 2006)

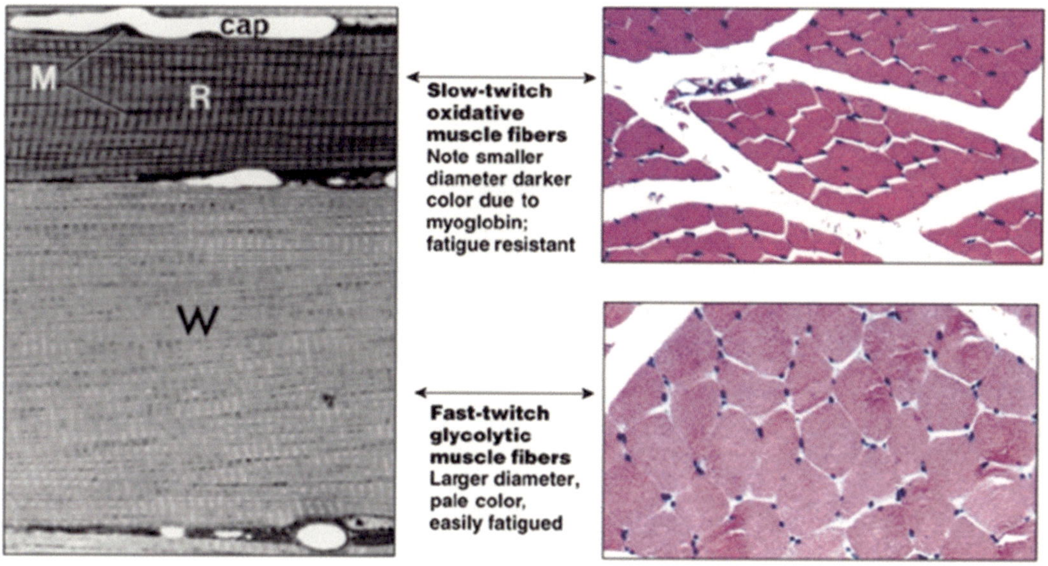

Fig. 1. Representative photographies to compare oxidative fibres to glycolytic fibres. On the left, there is a representative electron photomicrographs. On the right, muscles are stained with Haematoxylin-eosin (*source: Pearson education, Inc., publishing as Benjamin Cummings*).

Oxidative capacity of a given muscle can be linked to quantitative characteristics, especially mitochondrial and enzymatic contents. According to the relative importance of glycolysis and mitochondria, preferred substrate utilization can also vary from mainly carbohydrate to high-lipid utilization in highly oxidative muscles (Jackman & Willis, 1996; Ponsot et al., 2005).

Two families of muscles have been described in function of their metabolic activities. In oxidative muscles, composed essentially with slow oxidative fibres, the energy supplied continuously by mitochondria can sustain contractile activity for long periods of time without fatigue. By contrast, the glycolytic muscle composed with fast glycolytic fibres, has high levels of phosphocreatine and a high sensitivity to cytosolic ADP, which is, thus, the likely metabolic signal driving mitochondrial respiration (Mettauer et al., 2006).

Among these systems, there is the family of creatine kinase (CK) that catalyzes the reversible transfer of a phosphate moiety between creatine and adenosine diphosphate (ADP) (Mettauer et al., 2006). Four different isoforms of CK are expressed in a tissue specific and developmentally regulated manner. Among these isoforms, there is the mitochondrial isoenzyme (mi-CK), which is functionally coupled to oxidative phosphorylation and controls respiration in oxidative muscles (Wyss et al., 1992; Saks et al., 1994).

Mechanisms of high-energy phosphate transfer from mitochondria to local ATPases in the oxidative muscle fibres (type I skeletal muscle fibres, cardiac myocyte) can be described as "pay as you go" energy production, whereby, production is finely tuned to the needs of local ATPases within subcellular energetic units (figure 2).

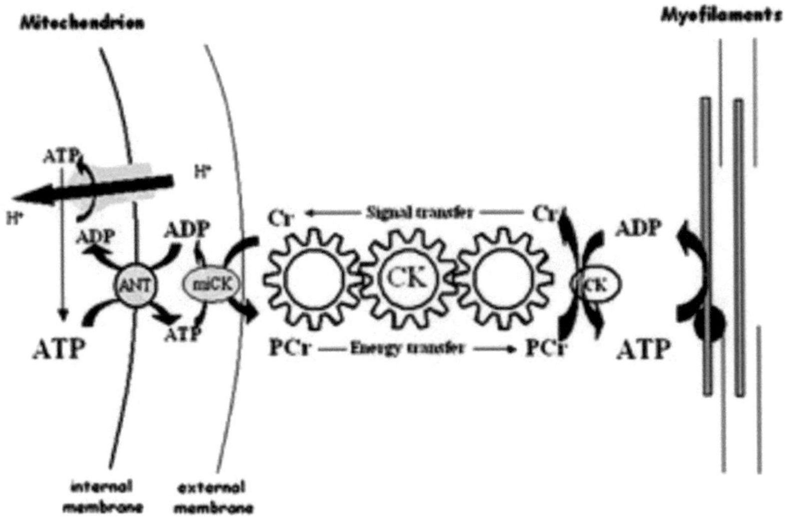

Fig. 2. The mechanisms of energy production in oxidative muscles, from. (Mettauer et al., 2006)

In glycolytic muscle fibres (type IIX/B), the mitochondria, together with glycolytic complexes, are concerned with replenishing intracellular phosphocreatine (PCr) stores which are immediately available for the ATPases-bound creatine kinases. This can be described as a "twitch now pay later" mode of operation (Kaasik et al., 2003; Ventura-Clapier et al., 2004; Mettauer et al., 2006)(figure 3).

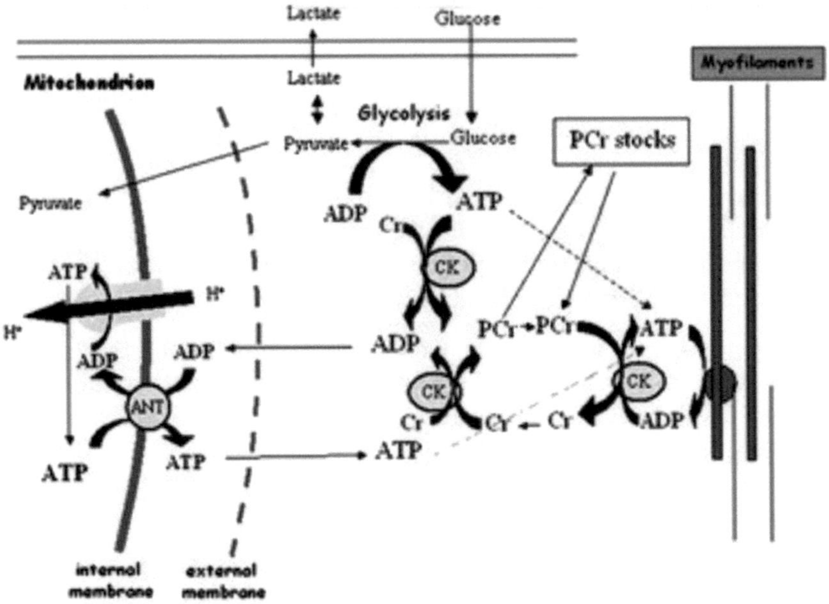

Fig. 3. The mechanisms of energy production in glycolytic muscles described before. (Mettauer et al., 2006)

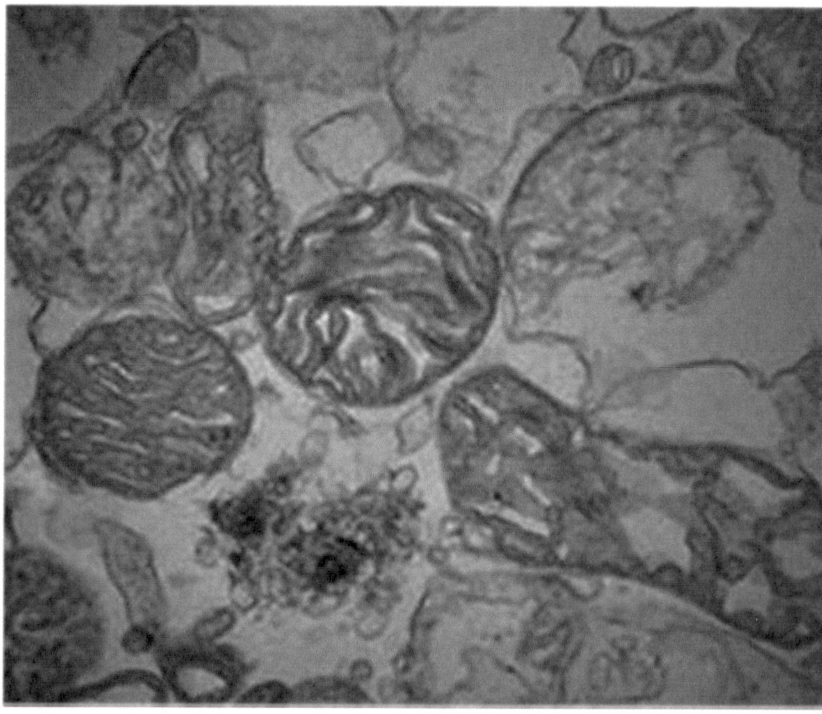

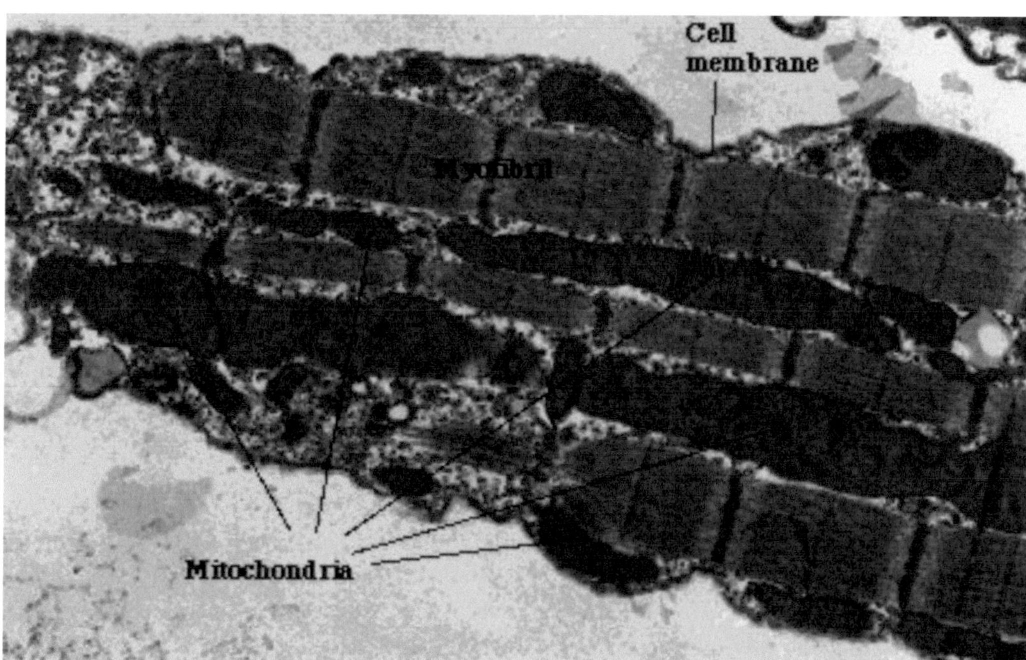

Fig. 4. Representative electron photomicrographs of mitochondrial ultrastructure in muscle fibres control (Mariappan et al., 2007). The second photo represents a muscle fibre with myofibrils and mitochondria (source: David R. Caprette, Rice University)

3. Mitochondrial analysis of muscle biopsy

3.1 Methods

Techniques and protocols of assessment of mitochondrial properties are of important physiological and physiopathological significance. 31P NMR spectroscopy has given the opportunity to study in vivo the intracellular metabolism under various conditions, including exercise in normal subjects and patients. However this approach did not reveal the intrinsic mitochondrial properties but rather the mitochondrial function under an uncontrolled intracellular medium. In the past, muscle mitochondrial properties were more closely explored either:

- By morphometric methods that give access to the mitochondria volume density and surface of cristae. The technique used the transmission electronic microscopy (figure 4) (Veksler et al., 1987),
- By biochemical methods determining the activity of intramitochondrial enzymes like citrate synthase (CS) and cytochrome oxidase (Cox). Actually, we can measure, directly the enzymatic activity of citrate synthase, which can be a good marker for quantifying mitochondria. Moreover, there are more and more different enzyme immunoassays to detect the consequence of the activities of metabolic enzymes. In addition, the different complexes implicated in the mitochondrial respiration can be explored (Birch-Machin & Turnbull, 2001).
- By polarographic methods, measuring O2 uptake of isolated mitochondria. These studies, on isolated mitochondria, required large amounts of tissue (approximately 500 mg), above the yield of routine human biopsy technique (10–50 mg), although efforts have been made to improve their sensitivity. More than two decades ago, Veksler et al. (Veksler et al., 1987) reported a method to assess the mitochondrial function of animal as well as human muscles. This new technique was based on the selective permeabilization of the sarcolemma by a low concentration of saponin (Kuznetsov et al., 2008). This approach allows the analysis of mitochondria within an integrated cellular system, preserving essential interactions with the cytoskeleton (Saks et al., 1998; Milner et al., 2000), nucleus (Dzeja et al., 2002) and endoplasmic reticulum (Rizzuto et al., 1998; Csordas et al., 2006).

3.2 Mitochondrial respiration

Oxidative phosphorylation has to be studied in intact mitochondria, which can be achieved by measuring the oxygen consumption of isolated mitochondria or muscle fibres from a tissue.

The skinned muscle fibre technique is adapted by Veksler and Saks for cardiac muscle fibres and also for skeletal muscle fibres (Veksler et al., 1987; Kuznetsov et al., 2008). This approach applies the ability of several chemical agents to specifically interact with the cholesterol in plasma membranes of cells or muscle fibres. These agents, for example saponin, have a high affinity to cholesterol and thus preferentially interact with cholesterol from membranes. Since, plasma membranes contain more cholesterol than the membrane of endoplasmic reticulum (ER) as well as the mitochondrial outer and inner membranes (Comte et al., 1976; Kuznetsov et al., 2008), there are no lesions on the intracellular membrane structures (mitochondria and ER) (Saks et al., 1998). Importantly, functionally intact mitochondria, myofilaments or sarcoplasmic reticulum (SR) of permeabilized muscle fibres respond quickly to changes in concentrations of ions, adenine nucleotides, substrates, inhibitors (Kuznetsov et al., 2008). So the intracellular space of permeabilized muscle fibres is equilibrated with the external medium (figure 5) (Veksler et al., 1987; Kunz et al., 1993; Kuznetsov et al., 1997; Kuznetsov et al., 1998; Kuznetsov et al., 2004), and mitochondria are able to use substrates added in the extracellular medium.

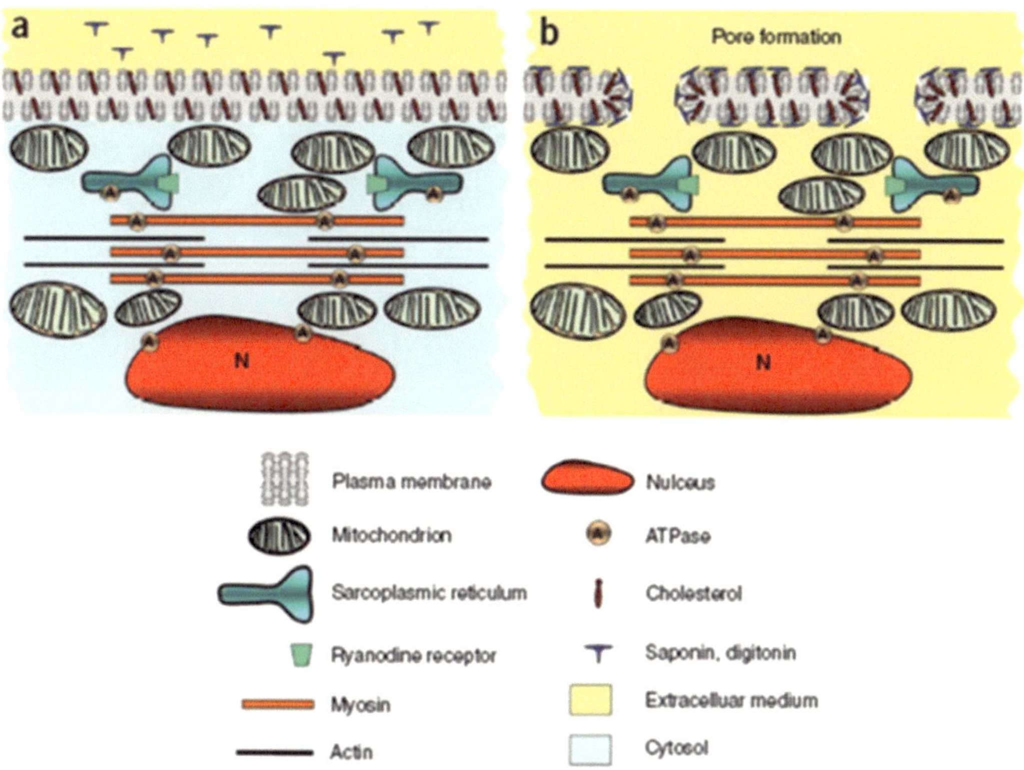

Fig. 5. Scheme explaining the effect of saponin on muscle fibres. Panel A represents the intracellular compartiment, with mitochondria, sarcoplasmic reticulum, nucleus (N). Panel B, when saponin acted; It appears a loss of plasmic membrane integrity. The mitochondrial sarcoplasmic membranes stayed intact. (Kuznetsov et al., 2008)

The addition of substrates allows us to analyze separately the different complexes I, II, III and IV of the mitochondrial respiratory chain. The measure consists in measuring the oxygen consumption polarographically with a Clark-type electrode. The substrates used are in function of the complex activity observed. The experiment started, all the time, by a measure of the basal respiration in non-phosphorylated condition but in the presence of glutamate-malate substrate, and is named V0. Then, for observing the maximal mitochondrial respiration by activating complexes I, III and IV, the addition of ADP (in saturating concentration) is sufficient, and the respiration rate is named Vmax. The next step is to activate the complex II in adding amytal or rotenone, (specific inhibitors of complex I), followed by the addition of succinate, this respiration rate is named Vsucc. The complex III can be inhibited by the addition of antimycin A. Finally, to measure the specific activity of complex IV, N, N, N', N'-tetramethyl-p-phenylenediamine dihydrochloride (TMPD) and ascorbate were added as an artificial electron donor to complex IV, the mitochondrial rate is named VTMPD/asc (Charles et al., 2011.; Kuznetsov et al., 2008)(figure 6).

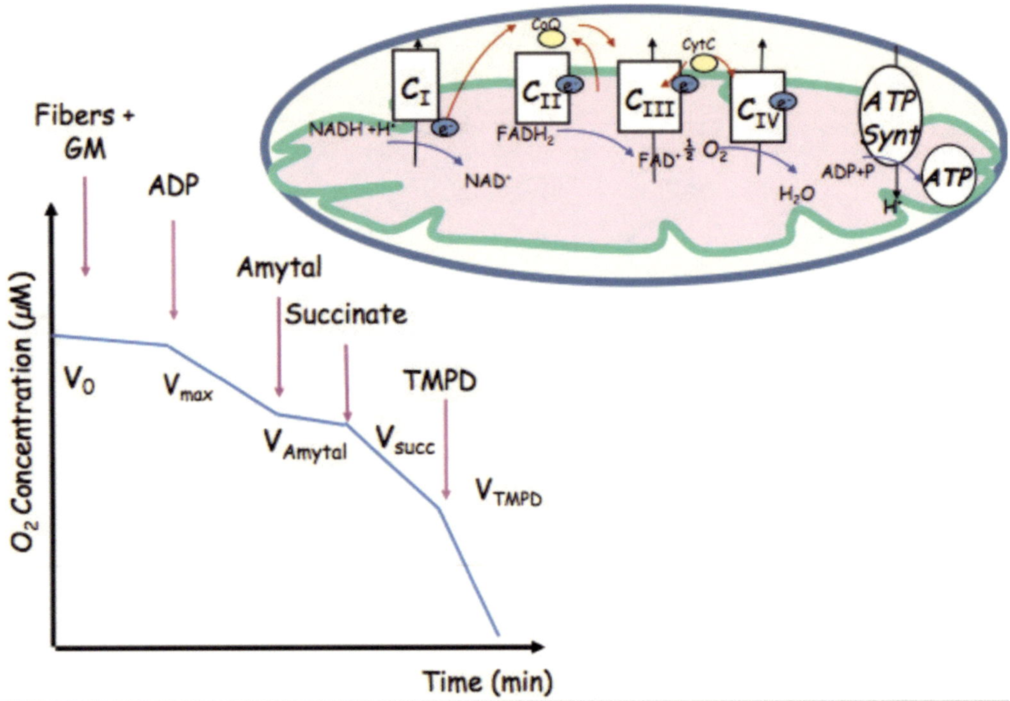

Fig. 6. Mitochondrial respiratory chain complexes activities using saponin skinned fibres. GM : glutamate/ malate. C_I: complex I; C_{II}: complex II; C_{III}: complex III ; C_{IV}: complex IV ; ATP Synt : ATP synthase ; cytC : cytochrome c; CoQ : coenzyme Q.

It is important to indicate that substrate utilization differ among muscle types (Baldwin et al., 1972; Holloszy & Booth, 1976; Jackman & Willis, 1996; Dyck et al., 1997). This means that muscle tissue has developed specific adaptations in terms of respiration control and intracellular energy distribution depending on its specific needs (Saks et al., 2001).

The Glycerol-3-Phosphate (G3-P) has a key role in the transfer of reducing equivalents from the cytosol to the mitochondrial matrix. This substrate is more used by the glycolytic muscles (Jackman & Willis, 1996).

Pyruvate is the substrate preferentially oxidized by all the different muscles (Ponsot et al., 2005). While the fatty acids like palmitoyl-carnitin are predominantly used by the cardiac and more generally by the oxidative skeletal muscles (Ponsot et al., 2005). The mechanisms of these different substrates are summarized in the figure 7.

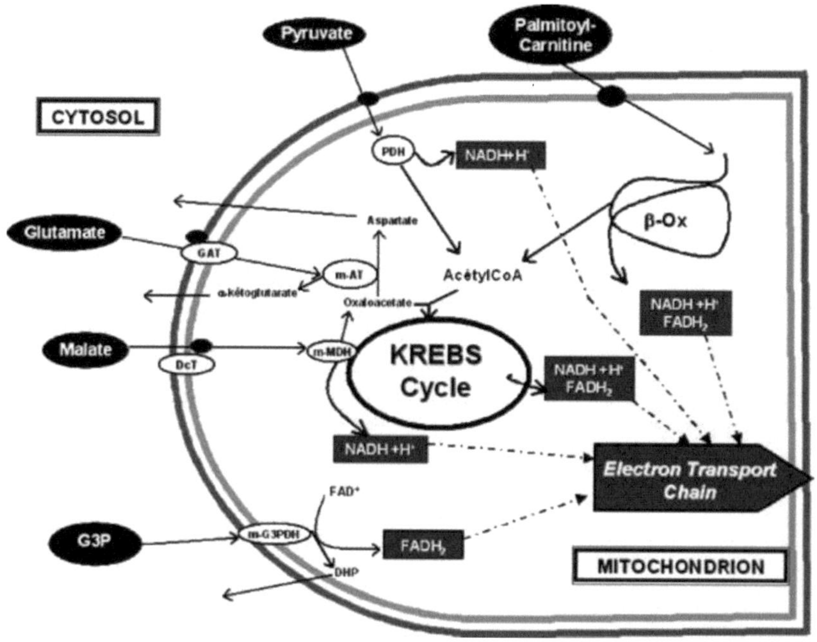

Fig. 7. The intervention of different substrates depending on their transport mechanism (Ponsot et al., 2005).
(1) pyruvate (Pyr), which activates the pyruvate dehydrogenase complex (PDH) localized in the mitochondrial matrix; (2) palmitoyl-carnitine (Palm-C), which is transferred into the matrix by the inner membrane-localized carnitine translocase (CT) and carnitine palmitoyl transferase II (CPTII), and activates the b-oxidation (b-ox); (3) G3-P, which diffuses to the intermembrane space and activates the mitochondrial G3-P dehydrogenase; (4) lactate (Lact), which could be converted into Pyr by mitochondrial LDH if it is present and functional. dicarboxylate translocase (DcT); dihydroxiacetone- phosphate (DHP); glutamate aspartate translocase (GAT); glycerol-3-phosphate (G3P); mitochondrial aspartate transaminase (m-AT); mitochondrial glycerol-3-phosphate dehydrogenase (m-G3PDH); mitochondrial malate dehydrogenase (m-MDH); pyruvate dehydrogenase complex (PDH).

3.3 Adenosine-5'-triphosphate (ATP) production

3.3.1 Definition

Adenosine-5'-triphosphate (ATP) is a multifunctional nucleotide used in cells as a coenzyme. ATP transports chemical energy within cells for metabolism. It is produced from Adenosine-5'-triphosphate (ADP) during glycolysis and the oxidative phosphorylation via the mitochondrial electron transport chain, which is the principal source of ATP in aerobic condition in mammals. ATP is used by enzymes and structural proteins in many cellular processes. It is used as a substrate in signal transduction pathways by kinases that phosphorylate proteins and lipids, as well as by Adenylate cyclase, which uses ATP to produce the second messenger molecule cyclic AMP. Apart from its roles in energy metabolism and signaling, ATP is also incorporated into nucleic acids by polymerases in the processes of DNA replication and transcription.

In muscle, it plays a crucial role for the contraction. Indeed, ATP is the direct energy source for muscle contraction (Rayment et al., 1993).

3.3.2 The interest of ATP measurement

In living cells, the distribution of ATP is ubiquitous, and is lost rapidly in dead cells. It is an appropriate marker for cell viability (Petty et al., 1995). Moreover ATP is extracted and measured easily.

3.3.3 Methods

Several methods exist allowing to quantify ATP concentration in myocytes:

- High-performance liquid chromatography (HPLC) with phosphate buffer as the mobile phase and UV detection (Lazzarino et al., 2003),
- Ion exchange chromatography, also with UV detection (Ally & Park, 1992; Maguire et al., 1992).
- However, the firefly luciferin-luciferase bioluminescence method is the most rapid, sensitive, and reproducible assay.

The bioluminescence assay is based on the reaction of ATP with recombinant firefly luciferase and its substrate luciferin. The stabilities of the reaction mixture as well as relevant ATP standards were quantified (Wibom & Hultman, 1990; Wibom et al., 1990).

It is a reagent based upon firefly luciferase, which emits light proportional to the ATP concentration.

The production of light is caused by the reaction of ATP with added luciferase and D-luciferin. This is illustrated in the following reaction scheme:

$$\text{ATP} + \text{D-Luciferin} + \text{O2} \xrightarrow[\text{Mg2+}]{\text{LUCIFERASE}} \text{Oxyluciferin} + \text{AMP} + \text{PPi} + \text{CO2} + \text{Light}$$

So, the ATP measurement permits to explain the importance of understanding the energy capacity of mitochondria in biology, physiology, cellular dysfunction, and ultimately, disease pathologies and aging (Drew & Leeuwenburgh, 2003; Aas et al., 2010).

3.4 Uncoupling of mitochondria

To phosphorylate ADP into ATP, the mitochondrion uses a coupling of oxidative phosphorylation across the mitochondrial inner membrane. But there is a phenomenon called mild uncoupling which allows the return of protons into the matrix without ATP production. This proton leak lowers the membrane potential across the inner membrane and increases the mitochondrial respiration rate (Brand, 1990). This leak goes by the uncoupling proteins (UCP). Discovered in 1978 (Nicholls et al., 1978), the first one, UCP1, localized in brown adipose tissue, is involved in cold-induced thermogenesis. The role of the other UCP, principally UCP2 (expressed ubiquitously) and UCP3 (expressed almost exclusively in skeletal muscle), is more controversial. As they are activated in extreme conditions (fasting, intensive exercise, high fat diet…) they could be a protective mechanism against oxidative stress. Indeed, when uncoupling is activated, mitochondrial respiration has to increase in order to maintain the membrane potential and ATP production. It seems that this mechanism reduces mitochondrial ROS production (Starkov, 1997).

Visualization of this phenomenon is indirect in vivo (calorimetric approaches), and only observed in vitro in specific conditions. The proton leak is shown from the measurement of the membrane potential together with the respiration rate (in non-phosphorylating state) (Brand, 1995; Cadenas et al., 2002).

3.5 ROS production

Reactive oxygen species (ROS) are involved in the regulation of many physiological processes. However, overproduction of ROS under various cellular stresses results in cell death and organ injury and thus contributes to a broad spectrum of diseases and pathological conditions. ROS are formed preferentially in mitochondria also under normal conditions and may participate in many signaling and regulation pathways. However, under various cell stresses, such as ischemia–reperfusion, hypoxia–reoxygenation, and treatment with toxic agents, mitochondrial ROS are produced in excess and are rapidly released into cytoplasm, where they may have damaging effects, leading to oxidative stress and cell injury. Different methods exist allowing to characterise ROS formation at the level of muscle tissue (see the chapter from Lejay et al. for much more explanations and the description of the methods).

3.6 Mitochondrial biogenesis and genes expression

Gene expression profiling is considered as a key technology for understanding the biology of tissue plasticity as well as pathological disorders. A growing body of evidence is accumulating that implies muscular gene expressional alterations to be involved to a significant extent in the unique response of cells and tissues to external stressors. Transcriptional profiling evolves as a powerful tool to explore the molecular mechanisms underlying such adaptation. Real time RT-PCR (reverse transcription-polymerase chain reation) is the basic but efficient technique allowing to explore mitochondrial gene expression in muscle.

Advances in molecular biology have started to elucidate the transcriptional events governing mitochondrial biogenesis. Peroxisome proliferator-activated receptor gamma co-activator (PGC-1α) is considered to be the major regulator of mitochondrial biogenesis (Ventura-Clapier et al., 2008). Mitochondrial biogenesis can be defined as the growth and division of pre-existing mitochondria. According to the accepted endosymbiotic theory, mitochondria are the direct descendants of a-proteobacteria endosymbiont that became established in a host cell. Due to their ancient bacterial origin, mitochondria have their own genome and a capacity for auto-replication. Mitochondrial proteins are encoded by the nuclear and the mitochondrial genomes. The double-strand circular mitochondrial DNA (mtDNA) is $\approx$16.5 kb in vertebrates and contains 37 genes encoding 13 subunits of the electron transport chain (ETC) complexes I, III, IV, and V, 22 transfer RNAs, and 2 ribosomal RNAs necessary for the translation. Correct mitochondrial biogenesis relies on the spatiotemporally coordinated synthesis and import of $\approx$1000 proteins encoded by the nuclear genome, of which some are assembled with proteins encoded by mitochondrial DNA within newly synthesized phospholipid membranes of the inner and outer mitochondrial membranes. All of these processes have to be tightly regulated in order to meet the tissue requirements. Mitochondrial biogenesis is triggered by environmental stresses such as exercise, cold exposure, caloric restriction, oxidative stress, cell division and renewal, and differentiation. The biogenesis of mitochondria is accompanied by variations in mitochondrial size, number, and mass. The discovery that alterations in mitochondrial biogenesis contribute to some chronic pathologies have increased the interest of the scientific community in this process and its regulation (Ventura-Clapier et al., 2008). Mitochondrial biogenesis is induced as followed: Peroxisome proliferator-activated receptor gamma co-activator (PGC-1a) activates nuclear transcription factors (NTFs) leading to transcription of nuclear-encoded proteins and of the mitochondrial transcription factor Tfam. Tfam activates transcription and replication of the mitochondrial genome. Nuclear-encoded proteins are imported into mitochondria through the outer- (TOM) or inner (TIM) membrane transport machinery. Nuclear- and mitochondria-encoded subunits of the respiratory chain are then assembled. Mitochondria in the cells of most tissues are tubular, and dynamic changes in morphology are driven by fission, fusion, and translocation (Bereiter-Hahn, 1990). The ability to undergo fission/fusion enables mitochondria to divide and helps ensure proper organization of the mitochondrial network during biogenesis. Mitochondrial fission is driven by dynamin-related proteins (DRP1 and OPA1), while mitochondrial fusion is controlled by mitofusins (Mfn1 and 2) (figure 8).

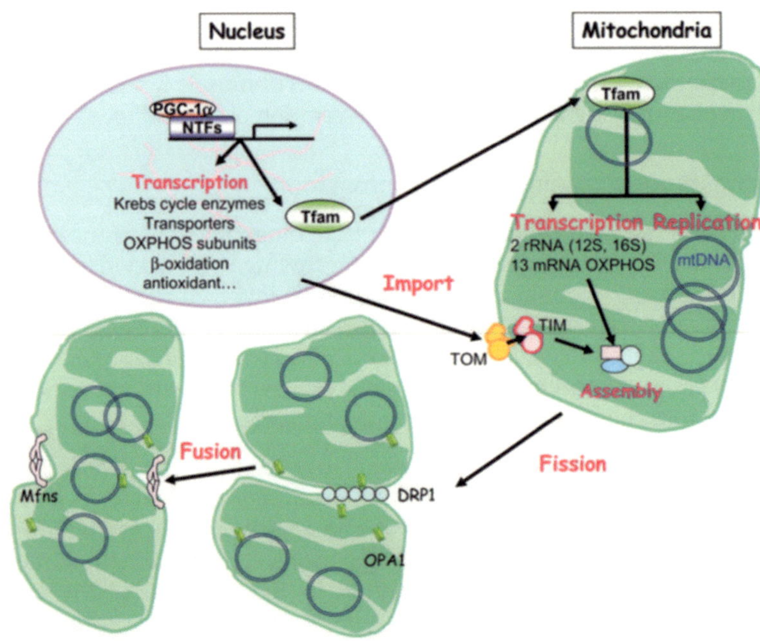

Fig. 8. Schematic representation of mitochondrial biogenesis. Peroxisome proliferator-activated receptor gamma co-activator (PGC-1α) activates nuclear transcription factors (NTFs) leading to transcription of nuclear- encoded proteins and of the mitochondrial transcription factor Tfam. Tfam activates transcription and replication of the mitochondrial genome. Nuclear-encoded proteins are imported into mitochondria through the outer- (TOM) or inner (TIM) membrane transport machinery. Nuclear- and mitochondria-encoded subunits of the respiratory chain are then assembled. Mitochondrial fission through the dynamin-related protein 1 (DRP1) for the outer membrane and OPA1 for the inner membrane of mitochondria allow mitochondrial division while mitofusins (Mfn) control mitochondrial fusion. Processes of fusion/fission lead to proper organization of the mitochondrial network. OXPHOS: oxidative phosphorylation (Ventura-Clapier *et al.*, 2008).

Measurement of mRNA expression of all theses proteins by RT-PCR technique could be a good means in order to show activation or deactivation of the mechanisms of mitochondrial biogenesis as well as mitochondrial fission/fusion. For details see the review of Ventura-Clapier et al (Ventura-Clapier et al., 2008).

In skeletal muscles, the consequences of a dysregulation of the mitochondrial biogenesis mechanisms could induce some important energetic changes including:

- a reduction of oxidative capacity and energy production;
- a decrease of energy transfer by the phosphotransfer kinases,
- a reduction of antioxidant buffering capacity;
- a global decrease of energy consumption efficiency. On the other hand, the signalling and molecular origins of these defects are unknown.

4. Analysis of muscle biopsy for detection of mitochondrial defects

Metabolic myopathies are inborn errors of metabolism that result in impaired energy production due to defects in glycogen, lipid, mitochondria, and possibly adenine nucleotide metabolism. Mitochondrial myopathies, fatty acid oxidation defects, and glycogen storage disease represent the three main groups of disorders (Burr et al., 2008; van Adel & Tarnopolsky, 2009). The mitochondrial myopathies manifest predominantly during endurance-type activity, under fasted or other metabolically stressful conditions. The clinical examination is often normal, and testing requires various combinations of exercise stress testing, serum creatine kinase activity and lactate concentration determination, urine organic acids, muscle biopsy, neuroimaging, and specific genetic testing for the diagnosis of a specific metabolic myopathy. Mitochondrial diseases are often disorders caused by an impairment of the mitochondrial respiratory chain function. They are usually progressive, isolated or multi-system diseases and have variable times of onset. Because mitochondria have their own DNA (mtDNA), mitochondrial diseases can be caused by mutations in both mtDNA and nuclear DNA (nDNA). The complexity of genetic control of mitochondrial function is in part responsible for the intra- and inter-familiar clinical heterogeneity of this class of diseases (Scarpelli et al., 2010).

Many forms of mitochondrial defects require a muscle biopsy to determine if any impairment exists. Unfortunately, not all mitochondrial defects are fully known, and so cannot be tested. Therefore, the detection of ragged red fibres by histological technique is looked for indications of a mitochondrial defect. A high lactic acid level is also often an indication. Moreover if a patient has three or more body systems affected, (for example circulatory, respiratory, and digestive systems), there is a suspicion of mitochondrial defect.

5. Skeletal muscle responses to metabolic and mechanical stimulations (i.e. physical exercise)

The introduction of the skeletal muscle biopsy procedure in the 1860's (Duchennes, 1864) has led to a tremendous step forward in our understanding of skeletal muscle physiology in humans. One of the fields that has most benefited from this new technique is the area of exercise physiology. There are major advances in the cellular and molecular mechanisms underlying the skeletal muscle responses to acute and chronic exercise, either with or without the combined effect of additional environmental stressors such as altitude or hypo/hyperthermia. Then, the skeletal muscle biopsy is considered as a masterpiece in the ongoing development of the integrative approach of exercise physiology. This links the molecular and cellular events occurring in individual skeletal muscle fibres to cellular, tissue and whole body structures and functions. Thanks to the insights provided by skeletal muscle biopsies, skeletal muscle plasticity to exercise training is currently believed to be driven by metabolic (i.e increased energy demand) or mechanical (i.e increased muscle tension) stimuli generated during the training sessions (Coyle, 2000; Dufour et al., 2007). The paragraphs below present some examples of scientific advances obtained through the use of skeletal muscle biopsies in the area of exercise physiology.

5.1 Skeletal muscle responses to metabolic stimulation

One way to selectively increase the metabolic stimulation on skeletal muscle is to compare normoxic vs hypoxic exercise training (Dufour, 2005). The lowered partial pressure for oxygen (PO2) in the inspired air translates into lowered muscle intracellular PO2 (Richardson et al., 1995), thereby triggering skeletal muscle adaptations to cope with the enhanced metabolic load. After 6 weeks of intermittent hypoxic vs normoxic treadmill training, our laboratory has shown specific and significant improvement in whole body aerobic performance capacity in endurance athletes (VO2max, time to exhaustion,...) (Dufour et al., 2006). Using biopsies of the vastus lateralis, we observed that the enhanced performance capacity was concomitant to an improved skeletal muscle mitochondrial function (Ponsot et al., 2006) and an up-regulated transcription of selected genes involved in oxygen sensing, mitochondrial biogenesis, mitochondrial metabolism, carbohydrate metabolism, pH regulation and oxidative stress (Zoll et al., 2006a). In this series of studies, muscle biopsies proved useful in highlighting the role of metabolic stimulations in the regulation of the metabolic component of skeletal muscle plasticity to exercise training.

5.2 Skeletal muscle responses to mechanical stimulation

Similarly to the metabolic stimuli, it is also possible to selectively increase the mechanical stimuli generated during the training sessions using concentric vs eccentric cycle ergometry (Dufour, 2005). Eccentric muscle actions are characterized by high forces and low energy expenditure emphasizing muscle mechanical tension with very little energy demand (Lastayo et al., 1999; Lastayo et al., 2000; Lindstedt et al., 2001; LaStayo et al., 2003b). Currently taken as a promising tool to develop skeletal muscle force in order to improve performance in athletes (Gross et al., 2010), eccentric cycle ergometry is also increasingly considered as a valuable method to counteract the impairment of skeletal muscle function observed in various populations including elderly (Lastayo et al., 2002; LaStayo et al., 2003a; LaStayo et al., 2007), chronic obstructive pulmonary disease (Rooyackers et al., 2003), coronary artery disease (Steiner et al., 2004), type 2 diabetes mellitus (Marcus et al., 2008; Marcus et al., 2009), Parkinson disease (Dibble et al., 2006a; Dibble et al., 2006b; Dibble et al., 2009), multiple sclerosis patients (Hayes et al., 2011) and cancer survivors (Hansen et al., 2009; Lastayo et al., 2010; LaStayo et al., 2011). After 8 weeks of eccentric vs concentric cycle ergometry with coronary patients, significant improvement in knee extensor muscle force has been observed (Steiner et al., 2004). Biopsies of vastus lateralis demonstrated an increased volume of myofibrils, an increased proportion of type IIa muscle fibres and an enhanced transcription of IGF-1 in the eccentric group (Zoll et al., 2006b). For the elderly patients (mean age = 80 yr old), eccentric cycle ergometry induced a greater gain in isometric strength of the knee extensors (Mueller et al., 2009), as compared with a conventional resistance training program. In this study, biopsies of vastus lateralis showed an enhanced expression of transcripts encoding factors involved in muscle growth, repair and remodeling (i.e. IGF-1, HGF, MYOG, MYH3) (Mueller et al., 2011). Of note, eccentric cycle ergometry was observed to depress genes encoding mitochondrial and metabolic transcripts. Taken together, the above experiments using muscle biopsies in human subjects show that mechanical stimulation of skeletal muscle trigger beneficial responses of the mechanical but not the metabolic component of skeletal muscle plasticity to exercise training.

5.3 Future developments in the muscle biopsy procedure

In human subjects, the withdrawal of muscle samples to perform biochemical, histochemical and histomorphometric muscle analyses has evolved from open air to semi open procedures (Henriksson, 1979), including "forceps" and the nowadays "gold standard" percutaneous Bergstrom needle procedure (Bergstrom, 1962). A suction system through the cutting trocard was introduced in 1982 in order to augment the size of the muscle tissue withdrawn at each insertion of the needle. These techniques do all need skin, subcutaneous and deep fascia anesthesia as well as a 5-10mm incision to access the muscle tissue with a 4 to 6 mm diameter Bergstrom needle (Hennessey et al., 1997). With these techniques, muscle samples of 77-170 mg can be obtained for each sample and doubling the sampling by rotating the needle 90° clockwise increased the size of the muscle sample to 172-271 mg in one pass (Hennessey et al., 1997). However, limitations exist for these procedures as their invasive character makes difficult the realization of serial sampling for studies examining the time course of intracellular physiological events (Hayot et al., 2005). Moreover, the procedure is sometimes difficult to get accepted by local ethics committee when applied to healthy normal subjects or athletes. Finally, some reservations should be made about the sterilization process and particularly the risk associated to Prion-contaminated medical instruments (sterilization of a hollow needle) (Weber & Rutala, 2002). As a less invasive alternative, microbiopsy procedures have been developed using fine disposable needles to obtain muscle samples in human subjects (Cote et al., 1992; Hayot et al., 2005). Although local anaesthesia is still required, skin incision is not always necessary. The skin is directly punctured with an insertion cannula perpendicular to the muscle until the fascia is pierced. The biopsy needle is subsequently inserted through the cannula and the muscle sample is obtained by the activation of a trigger button, which unloads the spring of the microbiopsy system and activates the needle to collect the muscle sample. Given the smaller size of the cannula and biopsy needles ranging from 11 to 18 gauges (i.e. 3.2 to 1.2 mm), the muscle samples obtained with microbiopsy procedures are much smaller. Despite the reduced muscle volumes, these developing microbiopsy procedures greatly facilitate serial muscle sampling either to increase the total size of the biopsy sample and/or to investigate the time course of intracellular physiological process of interest. An additional strength of the microbiopsy is that the procedure has been reported to be much more comfortable for the subjects and easier to perform compared to open air or percutaneous Bergstrom needle procedure (Cote et al., 1992; Hayot et al., 2005), allowing its wider use in the future of many areas of skeletal muscle physiology, including exercise physiology.

6. Conclusion

Exploration of energetic metabolism with skeletal muscle biopsy is central in order to characterise and to better understand the mitochondrial function and the mechanisms of cell death and pathophysiology of a variety of human diseases, including myopathies, neurodegenerative diseases, heart failure, diabetes and cancer. Indeed, clinical implications such as reduced exercise capacity, reduced quality of life are related to changes in muscle mitochondrial function. In the last decade, new experimental approaches with new biological techniques were applied to human biopsies allowing to help to diagnose several metabolic impairments in skeletal muscle. A lot of mitochondrial dysfunctions developed in chronic disease may be reversible, and then, improvement of the comprehension of mitochondrial physiology and pathophysiology could help to find new therapeutic avenues in the future.

7. References

(1999). Skeletal muscle dysfunction in chronic obstructive pulmonary disease. A statement of the American Thoracic Society and European Respiratory Society. *Am J Respir Crit Care Med* 159, S1-40.

Aas V, Hessvik NP, Wettergreen M, Hvammen AW, Hallen S, Thoresen GH & Rustan AC. (2010). Chronic hyperglycemia reduces substrate oxidation and impairs metabolic switching of human myotubes. *Biochim Biophys Acta* 1812, 94-105.

Ally A & Park G. (1992). Rapid determination of creatine, phosphocreatine, purine bases and nucleotides (ATP, ADP, AMP, GTP, GDP) in heart biopsies by gradient ion-pair reversed-phase liquid chromatography. *J Chromatogr* 575, 19-27.

Baldwin KM, Fitts RH, Booth FW, Winder WW & Holloszy JO. (1975). Depletion of muscle and liver glycogen during exercise. Protective effect of training. *Pflugers Arch* 354, 203-212.

Baldwin KM, Klinkerfuss GH, Terjung RL, Mole PA & Holloszy JO. (1972). Respiratory capacity of white, red, and intermediate muscle: adaptative response to exercise. *Am J Physiol* 222, 373-378.

Bereiter-Hahn J. (1990). Behavior of mitochondria in the living cell. *Int Rev Cytol* 122, 1-63.

Bergstrom J. (1962). Muscle electrolytes in humans. *Scand J Clin Lab Invest* 14, 511-513.

Birch-Machin MA & Turnbull DM. (2001). Assaying mitochondrial respiratory complex activity in mitochondria isolated from human cells and tissues. *Methods Cell Biol* 65, 97-117.

Brand MD. (1990). The proton leak across the mitochondrial inner membrane. *Biochim Biophys Acta* 1018, 128-133.

Brand MD. (1995). Bioenergetics: A pratical approach. In IRL Press, Oxford edn, ed. Brown GC, and Cooper, C.E., eds, pp. p39-62.

Burr ML, Roos JC & Ostor AJ. (2008). Metabolic myopathies: a guide and update for clinicians. *Curr Opin Rheumatol* 20, 639-647.

Cadenas S, Echtay KS, Harper JA, Jekabsons MB, Buckingham JA, Grau E, Abuin A, Chapman H, Clapham JC & Brand MD. (2002). The Basal Proton Conductance of Skeletal Muscle Mitochondria from Transgenic Mice Overexpressing or Lacking Uncoupling Protein-3. *J Biol Chem* 277, 2773-2778.

Charles AL, Guilbert AS, Bouitbir J, Goette-Di Marco P, Enache I, Zoll J, Piquard F & Geny B. Effect of postconditioning on mitochondrial dysfunction in experimental aortic cross-clamping. *Br J Surg* 98, 511-516.

Comte J, Maisterrena B & Gautheron DC. (1976). Lipid composition and protein profiles of outer and inner membranes from pig heart mitochondria. Comparison with microsomes. *Biochim Biophys Acta* 419, 271-284.

Cote AM, Jimenez L, Adelman LS & Munsat TL. (1992). Needle muscle biopsy with the automatic Biopty instrument. *Neurology* 42, 2212-2213.

Coyle EF. (2000). Physical activity as a metabolic stressor. *Am J Clin Nutr* 72, 512S-520S.

Csordas G, Renken C, Varnai P, Walter L, Weaver D, Buttle KF, Balla T, Mannella CA & Hajnoczky G. (2006). Structural and functional features and significance of the physical linkage between ER and mitochondria. *J Cell Biol* 174, 915-921.

De Sousa E, Veksler V, Bigard X, Mateo P & Ventura-Clapier R. (2000). Heart failure affects mitochondrial but not myofibrillar intrinsic properties of skeletal muscle. *Circulation* 102, 1847-1853.

Dibble LE, Hale T, Marcus RL, Gerber JP & Lastayo PC. (2006a). The safety and feasibility of high-force eccentric resistance exercise in persons with Parkinson's disease. *Arch Phys Med Rehabil* 87, 1280-1282.

Dibble LE, Hale TF, Marcus RL, Droge J, Gerber JP & LaStayo PC. (2006b). High-intensity resistance training amplifies muscle hypertrophy and functional gains in persons with Parkinson's disease. *Mov Disord* 21, 1444-1452.

Dibble LE, Hale TF, Marcus RL, Gerber JP & LaStayo PC. (2009). High intensity eccentric resistance training decreases bradykinesia and improves Quality Of Life in persons with Parkinson's disease: a preliminary study. *Parkinsonism Relat Disord* 15, 752-757.

Drew B & Leeuwenburgh C. (2003). Method for measuring ATP production in isolated mitochondria: ATP production in brain and liver mitochondria of Fischer-344 rats with age and caloric restriction. *Am J Physiol Regul Integr Comp Physiol* 285, R1259-1267.

Drexler H. (1992). Skeletal muscle failure in heart failure. *Circulation* 85, 1621-1623.

Duchennes GB. (1864). Recherches sur la paralysie musculaire pseudohypertrophique ou paralysie myosclérotique. *Archives Générales de Médecine* 11, 179.

Dufour SP. (2005). Optimisation de la performance aérobie chez l'athlète: hypoxie intermittente à l'exercice et ergocycle excentrique comme nouvelles méthodes de stimulation métabolique et mécanique. In *Institute of Physiology, Faculty of Medicine*. University of Strasbourg, Strasbourg.

Dufour SP, Doutreleau S, Lonsdorfer-Wolf E, Lampert E, Hirth C, Piquard F, Lonsdorfer J, Geny B, Mettauer B & Richard R. (2007). Deciphering the metabolic and mechanical contributions to the exercise-induced circulatory response: insights from eccentric cycling. *Am J Physiol Regul Integr Comp Physiol* 292, R1641-R1648.

Dufour SP, Ponsot E, Zoll J, Doutreleau S, Lonsdorfer-Wolf E, Geny B, Lampert E, Fluck M, Hoppeler H, Billat V, Mettauer B, Richard R & Lonsdorfer J. (2006). Exercise training in normobaric hypoxia in endurance runners. I. Improvement in aerobic performance capacity. *J Appl Physiol* 100, 1238-1248.

Dyck DJ, Peters SJ, Glatz J, Gorski J, Keizer H, Kiens B, Liu S, Richter EA, Spriet LL, van der Vusse GJ & Bonen A. (1997). Functional differences in lipid metabolism in resting skeletal muscle of various fiber types. *Am J Physiol* 272, E340-351.

Dzeja PP, Bortolon R, Perez-Terzic C, Holmuhamedov EL & Terzic A. (2002). Energetic communication between mitochondria and nucleus directed by catalyzed phosphotransfer. *Proc Natl Acad Sci U S A* 99, 10156-10161.

Fluck M & Hoppeler H. (2003). Molecular basis of skeletal muscle plasticity--from gene to form and function. *Rev Physiol Biochem Pharmacol* 146, 159-216.

Gross M, Luthy F, Kroell J, Muller E, Hoppeler H & Vogt M. (2010). Effects of eccentric cycle ergometry in alpine skiers. *Int J Sports Med* 31, 572-576.

Hambrecht R, Niebauer J, Fiehn E, Kalberer B, Offner B, Hauer K, Riede U, Schlierf G, Kubler W & Schuler G. (1995). Physical training in patients with stable chronic heart failure: effects on cardiorespiratory fitness and ultrastructural abnormalities of leg muscles. *J Am Coll Cardiol* 25, 1239-1249.

Hansen PA, Dechet CB, Porucznik CA & LaStayo PC. (2009). Comparing eccentric resistance exercise in prostate cancer survivors on and off hormone therapy: a pilot study. *PM R* 1, 1019-1024.

Hayes HA, Gappmaier E & LaStayo PC. (2011). Effects of high-intensity resistance training on strength, mobility, balance, and fatigue in individuals with multiple sclerosis: a randomized controlled trial. *J Neurol Phys Ther* 35, 2-10.

Hayot M, Michaud A, Koechlin C, Caron MA, Leblanc P, Prefaut C & Maltais F. (2005). Skeletal muscle microbiopsy: a validation study of a minimally invasive technique. *Eur Respir J* 25, 431-440.

Hennessey JV, Chromiak JA, Della Ventura S, Guertin J & MacLean DB. (1997). Increase in percutaneous muscle biopsy yield with a suction-enhancement technique. *J Appl Physiol* 82, 1739-1742.

Henriksson KG. (1979). "Semi-open" muscle biopsy technique. A simple outpatient procedure. *Acta Neurol Scand* 59, 317-323.

Holloszy JO & Booth FW. (1976). Biochemical adaptations to endurance exercise in muscle. *Annu Rev Physiol* 38, 273-291.

Jackman MR & Willis WT. (1996). Characteristics of mitochondria isolated from type I and type IIb skeletal muscle. *Am J Physiol* 270, C673-678.

Johannsen DL & Ravussin E. (2009). The role of mitochondria in health and disease. *Curr Opin Pharmacol* 9, 780-786.

Kaasik A, Veksler V, Boehm E, Novotova M & Ventura-Clapier R. (2003). From energy store to energy flux: a study in creatine kinase-deficient fast skeletal muscle. *FASEB J* 17, 708-710.

Kunz WS, Kuznetsov AV, Schulze W, Eichhorn K, Schild L, Striggow F, Bohnensack R, Neuhof S, Grasshoff H, Neumann HW & Gellerich FN. (1993). Functional characterization of mitochondrial oxidative phosphorylation in saponin-skinned human muscle fibers. *Biochim Biophys Acta* 1144, 46-53.

Kuznetsov AV, Mayboroda O, Kunz D, Winkler K, Schubert W & Kunz WS. (1998). Functional imaging of mitochondria in saponin-permeabilized mice muscle fibers. *J Cell Biol* 140, 1091-1099.

Kuznetsov AV, Schneeberger S, Seiler R, Brandacher G, Mark W, Steurer W, Saks V, Usson Y, Margreiter R & Gnaiger E. (2004). Mitochondrial defects and heterogeneous cytochrome c release after cardiac cold ischemia and reperfusion. *Am J Physiol Heart Circ Physiol* 286, H1633-1641.

Kuznetsov AV, Veksler V, Gellerich FN, Saks V, Margreiter R & Kunz WS. (2008). Analysis of mitochondrial function in situ in permeabilized muscle fibers, tissues and cells. *Nat Protoc* 3, 965-976.

Kuznetsov AV, Winkler K, Kirches E, Lins H, Feistner H & Kunz WS. (1997). Application of inhibitor titrations for the detection of oxidative phosphorylation defects in saponin-skinned muscle fibers of patients with mitochondrial diseases. *Biochim Biophys Acta* 1360, 142-150.

LaStayo P, McDonagh P, Lipovic D, Napoles P, Bartholomew A, Esser K & Lindstedt S. (2007). Elderly patients and high force resistance exercise--a descriptive report: can an anabolic, muscle growth response occur without muscle damage or inflammation? *J Geriatr Phys Ther* 30, 128-134.

LaStayo PC, Ewy GA, Pierotti DD, Johns RK & Lindstedt S. (2003a). The positive effects of negative work: increased muscle strength and decreased fall risk in a frail elderly population. *J Gerontol A Biol Sci Med Sci* 58, M419-424.

Lastayo PC, Johns R, McDonagh P & Lindstedt SL. (2002). High-force eccentric exercise for sarcopenia. *Med Sci Sports Exerc* 34 Suppl 1, p 6.

Lastayo PC, Larsen S, Smith S, Dibble L & Marcus R. (2010). The feasibility and efficacy of eccentric exercise with older cancer survivors: a preliminary study. *J Geriatr Phys Ther* 33, 135-140.

LaStayo PC, Marcus RL, Dibble LE, Smith SB & Beck SL. (2011). Eccentric exercise versus usual-care with older cancer survivors: the impact on muscle and mobility--an exploratory pilot study. *BMC Geriatr* 11, 5.

Lastayo PC, Pierotti DJ, Pifer J, Hoppeler H & Lindstedt SL. (2000). Eccentric ergometry: increases in locomotor muscle size and strength at low training intensities. *Am J Physiol Regul Integr Comp Physiol* 278, R1282-R1288.

Lastayo PC, Reich TE, Urquhart M, Hoppeler H & Lindstedt SL. (1999). Chronic eccentric exercise: improvements in muscle strength can occur with little demand for oxygen. *Am J Physiol* 276, R611-R615.

LaStayo PC, Woolf JM, Lewek MD, Snyder-Mackler L, Reich T & Lindstedt SL. (2003b). Eccentric muscle contractions: their contribution to injury, prevention, rehabilitation, and sport. *J Orthop Sports Phys Ther* 33, 557-571.

Lazzarino G, Amorini AM, Fazzina G, Vagnozzi R, Signoretti S, Donzelli S, Di Stasio E, Giardina B & Tavazzi B. (2003). Single-sample preparation for simultaneous cellular redox and energy state determination. *Anal Biochem* 322, 51-59.

Lindstedt SL, Lastayo PC & Reich TE. (2001). When active muscles lengthen: properties and consequences of eccentric contractions. *News Physiol Sci* 16, 256-261.

Maguire MH, Szabo I, Slegel P & King CR. (1992). Determination of concentrations of adenosine and other purines in human term placenta by reversed-phase high-performance liquid chromatography with photodiode-array detection: evidence for pathways of purine metabolism in the placenta. *J Chromatogr* 575, 243-253.

Maltais F, Simard AA, Simard C, Jobin J, Desgagnes P & LeBlanc P. (1996). Oxidative capacity of the skeletal muscle and lactic acid kinetics during exercise in normal subjects and in patients with COPD. *Am J Respir Crit Care Med* 153, 288-293.

Marcus RL, Lastayo PC, Dibble LE, Hill L & McClain DA. (2009). Increased strength and physical performance with eccentric training in women with impaired glucose tolerance: a pilot study. *J Womens Health (Larchmt)* 18, 253-260.

Marcus RL, Smith S, Morrell G, Addison O, Dibble LE, Wahoff-Stice D & Lastayo PC. (2008). Comparison of combined aerobic and high-force eccentric resistance exercise with aerobic exercise only for people with type 2 diabetes mellitus. *Phys Ther* 88, 1345-1354.

Mariappan N, Soorappan RN, Haque M, Sriramula S & Francis J. (2007). TNF-alpha-induced mitochondrial oxidative stress and cardiac dysfunction: restoration by superoxide dismutase mimetic Tempol. *Am J Physiol Heart Circ Physiol* 293, H2726-2737.

Mettauer B, Zoll J, Garnier A & Ventura-Clapier R. (2006). Heart failure: a model of cardiac and skeletal muscle energetic failure. *Pflugers Arch* 452, 653-666.

Mettauer B, Zoll J, Sanchez H, Lampert E, Ribera F, Veksler V, Bigard X, Mateo P, Epailly E, Lonsdorfer J & Ventura-Clapier R. (2001). Oxidative capacity of skeletal muscle in heart failure patients versus sedentary or active control subjects. *J Am Coll Cardiol* 38, 947-954.

Milner DJ, Mavroidis M, Weisleder N & Capetanaki Y. (2000). Desmin cytoskeleton linked to muscle mitochondrial distribution and respiratory function. *J Cell Biol* 150, 1283-1298.

Mueller M, Breil FA, Lurman G, Klossner S, Fluck M, Billeter R, Dapp C & Hoppeler H. (2011). Different Molecular and Structural Adaptations with Eccentric and Conventional Strength Training in Elderly Men and Women. *Gerontology*.

Mueller M, Breil FA, Vogt M, Steiner R, Lippuner K, Popp A, Klossner S, Hoppeler H & Dapp C. (2009). Different response to eccentric and concentric training in older men and women. *Eur J Appl Physiol* 107, 145-153.

Nicholls DG, Bernson VS & Heaton GM. (1978). The identification of the component in the inner membrane of brown adipose tissue mitochondria responsible for regulating energy dissipation. *Experientia Suppl* 32, 89-93.

Petty RD, Sutherland LA, Hunter EM & Cree IA. (1995). Comparison of MTT and ATP-based assays for the measurement of viable cell number. *J Biolumin Chemilumin* 10, 29-34.

Ponsot E, Dufour SP, Zoll J, Doutrelau S, N'Guessan B, Geny B, Hoppeler H, Lampert E, Mettauer B, Ventura-Clapier R & Richard R. (2006). Exercise training in normobaric hypoxia in endurance runners. II. Improvement of mitochondrial properties in skeletal muscle. *J Appl Physiol* 100, 1249-1257.

Ponsot E, Zoll J, N'Guessan B, Ribera F, Lampert E, Richard R, Veksler V, Ventura-Clapier R & Mettauer B. (2005). Mitochondrial tissue specificity of substrates utilization in rat cardiac and skeletal muscles. *J Cell Physiol* 203, 479-486.

Rayment I, Holden HM, Whittaker M, Yohn CB, Lorenz M, Holmes KC & Milligan RA. (1993). Structure of the actin-myosin complex and its implications for muscle contraction. *Science* 261, 58-65.

Richardson RS, Noyszewski EA, Kendrick KF, Leigh JS & Wagner PD. (1995). Myoglobin O2 desaturation during exercise. Evidence of limited O2 transport. *J Clin Invest* 96, 1916-1926.

Rizzuto R, Pinton P, Carrington W, Fay FS, Fogarty KE, Lifshitz LM, Tuft RA & Pozzan T. (1998). Close contacts with the endoplasmic reticulum as determinants of mitochondrial Ca2+ responses. *Science* 280, 1763-1766.

Rooyackers JM, Berkeljon DA & Folgering HT. (2003). Eccentric exercise training in patients with chronic obstructive pulmonary disease. *Int J Rehabil Res* 26, 47-49.

Saks VA, Kaambre T, Sikk P, Eimre M, Orlova E, Paju K, Piirsoo A, Appaix F, Kay L, Regitz-Zagrosek V, Fleck E & Seppet E. (2001). Intracellular energetic units in red muscle cells. *Biochem J* 356, 643-657.

Saks VA, Khuchua ZA, Vasilyeva EV, Belikova O & Kuznetsov AV. (1994). Metabolic compartmentation and substrate channelling in muscle cells. Role of coupled creatine kinases in in vivo regulation of cellular respiration--a synthesis. *Mol Cell Biochem* 133-134, 155-192.

Saks VA, Veksler VI, Kuznetsov AV, Kay L, Sikk P, Tiivel T, Tranqui L, Olivares J, Winkler K, Wiedemann F & Kunz WS. (1998). Permeabilized cell and skinned fiber techniques in studies of mitochondrial function in vivo. *Mol Cell Biochem* 184, 81-100.

Scarpelli M, Cotelli MS, Mancuso M, Tomelleri G, Tonin P, Baronchelli C, Vielmi V, Gregorelli V, Todeschini A, Padovani A & Filosto M. (2010). Current options in the treatment of mitochondrial diseases. *Recent Pat CNS Drug Discov* 5, 203-209.

Schiaffino S & Reggiani C. (1996). Molecular diversity of myofibrillar proteins: gene regulation and functional significance. *Physiol Rev* 76, 371-423.

Starkov AA. (1997). "Mild" uncoupling of mitochondria. *Biosci Rep* 17, 273-279.

Steiner R, Meyer K, Lippuner K, Schmid JP, Saner H & Hoppeler H. (2004). Eccentric endurance training in subjects with coronary artery disease: a novel exercise paradigm in cardiac rehabilitation? *Eur J Appl Physiol* 91, 572-578.

van Adel BA & Tarnopolsky MA. (2009). Metabolic myopathies: update 2009. *J Clin Neuromuscul Dis* 10, 97-121.

Veksler VI, Kuznetsov AV, Sharov VG, Kapelko VI & Saks VA. (1987). Mitochondrial respiratory parameters in cardiac tissue: a novel method of assessment by using saponin-skinned fibers. *Biochim Biophys Acta* 892, 191-196.

Ventura-Clapier R, Garnier A & Veksler V. (2008). Transcriptional control of mitochondrial biogenesis: the central role of PGC-1alpha. *Cardiovasc Res* 79, 208-217.

Ventura-Clapier R, Kaasik A & Veksler V. (2004). Structural and functional adaptations of striated muscles to CK deficiency. *Mol Cell Biochem* 256-257, 29-41.

Weber DJ & Rutala WA. (2002). Managing the risk of nosocomial transmission of prion diseases. *Curr Opin Infect Dis* 15, 421-425.

Wibom R & Hultman E. (1990). ATP production rate in mitochondria isolated from microsamples of human muscle. *Am J Physiol* 259, E204-209.

Wibom R, Lundin A & Hultman E. (1990). A sensitive method for measuring ATP-formation in rat muscle mitochondria. *Scand J Clin Lab Invest* 50, 143-152.

Williams AD, Selig S, Hare DL, Hayes A, Krum H, Patterson J, Geerling RH, Toia D & Carey MF. (2004). Reduced exercise tolerance in CHF may be related to factors other than impaired skeletal muscle oxidative capacity. *J Card Fail* 10, 141-148.

Wyss M, Smeitink J, Wevers RA & Wallimann T. (1992). Mitochondrial creatine kinase: a key enzyme of aerobic energy metabolism. *Biochim Biophys Acta* 1102, 119-166.

Zoll J, Ponsot E, Dufour S, Doutreleau S, Ventura-Clapier R, Vogt M, Hoppeler H, Richard R & Fluck M. (2006a). Exercise training in normobaric hypoxia in endurance runners. III. Muscular adjustments of selected gene transcripts. *J Appl Physiol* 100, 1258-1266.

Zoll J, Steiner R, Meyer K, Vogt M, Hoppeler H & Fluck M. (2006b). Gene expression in skeletal muscle of coronary artery disease patients after concentric and eccentric endurance training. *Eur J Appl Physiol* 96, 413-422.

Skeletal Muscle Mitochondrial Function in Peripheral Arterial Disease: Usefulness of Muscle Biopsy

A. Lejay, A.L. Charles, J. Zoll, J. Bouitbir,
F. Thaveau, F. Piquard and B. Geny
University of Strasbourg
France

1. Introduction

1.1 Peripheral arterial disease

Peripheral arterial disease (PAD) is a manifestation of atherosclerosis which produces stenoses and occlusions in lower limbs arteries. PAD was commonly divided in four stages, introduced by Rene Fontaine in 1954 (Fontaine *et al.*, 1954): stage 1 defined an asymptomatic patient, stage 2 defined a patient presenting with a significant impairment of his ability to walk (intermittent claudication). Then claudication worsens and the patient develops rest pain in stage 3, and non-healing ulcers or gangrene in stage 4.

Recently, other criteria have been proposed for the diagnosis of PAD. Stage 2 of Leriche is now called « functional ischemia », and stages 3 and 4 are now called « critical ischemia » (Norgren *et al.*, 2007). Critical ischemia is called this way because of its poor prognosis. With this new classification, the diagnosis of critical limb ischemia requires both clinical criteria, but also hemodynamic criteria (ankle-brachial index, toe pressure). Normal values of ankle-brachial index are between 0,9 and 1,3. PAD is characterized by ankle-brachial values under 0,9 (0,4-0,9: functional ischemia, <0,4: critical ischemia). The normal value of the toe pressure is 60-65 mm Hg, it can be normal or within the limits of the normal in functional ischemia, but it is commonly under 10 mm Hg in critical ischemia. These hemodynamic criteria objectify the arterial etiology of the lesions, because it is sometimes difficult to define the exact origin of rest pain or tissue loss (diabetes, venous insufficiency…).

Insufficient oxygen supply secondary to reduced blood flow is presumed to be the main physiologic cause for the manifestations of peripheral arterial disease, but more recently the presence of mitochondriopathy in chronically ischemic skeletal muscle has been proposed. Suboptimal energy production from defective mitochondria participates in PAD pathogenesis in addition to reduced oxygen supply (Marbini *et al.*, 1986; Lundgren *et al.*, 1989; Bhat *et al.*, 1999; Brass *et al.*, 2001; Pipinos *et al.*, 2008a)(Figure 1).

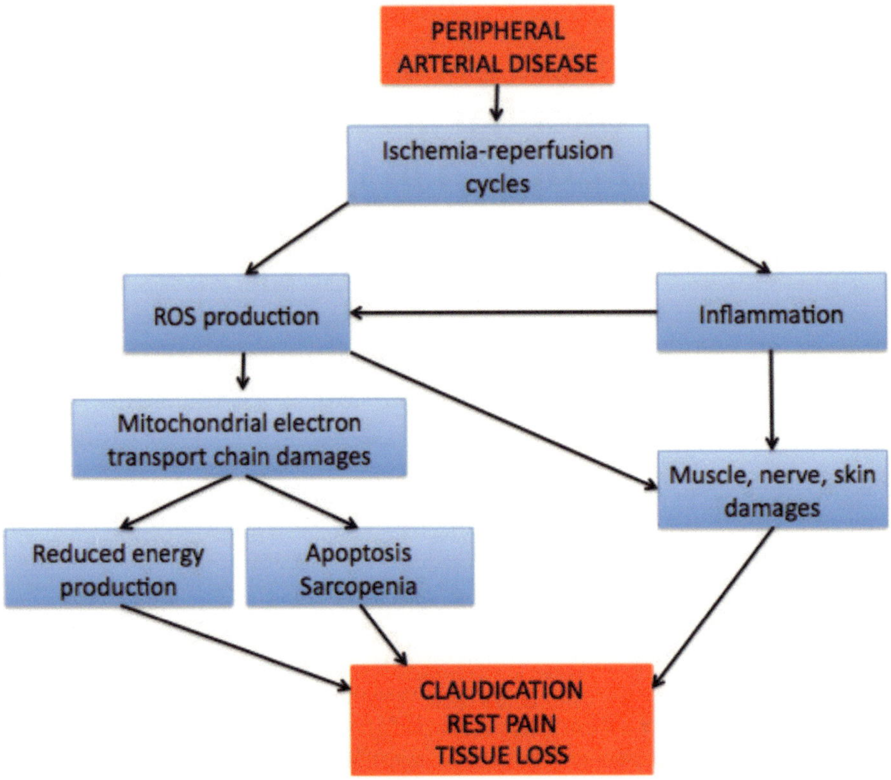

Fig. 1. Pathogenesis of peripheral arterial disease

1.2 Mitochondrial function and oxidative stress

Every action requires energy, and this energy is stored in adenosine triphosphate (ATP) molecules that are produced in the mitochondria by the process of oxidative phosphorylation. Mitochondria are present in every cell, but there are in high concentrations in muscle cells because high energetic requirements of muscles.

1.2.1 Structure of mitochondria

Mitochondria are enclosed within two membranes: the outer membrane and the inner membrane. The outer membrane is a relatively simple phospholipid bilayer, containing protein structures called porins which allow molecules of 10 kilodaltons in weight to pass through it. This explains why the outer membrane is completely permeable to nutrient molecules, ions, ATP and ADP molecules. The inner membrane is more complex in structure than the outer membrane because it contains electron transport chain, ATP synthetase, and transport proteins. It is freely permeable only to oxygen, carbon dioxide and water. The wrinkles, or folds, are organized into layers called cristae, which increase total surface area of the inner membrane (figure2).

Outer and inner membranes delineate two compartments: the intermembrane space, and the cytoplasmic matrix. The intermembrane space is located between the inner and the outer membranes. It has an important role in oxidative phosphorylation. The cytoplasmic matrix contains the enzymes that are responsible for citric acid cycle reactions. The matrix also contains dissolved oxygen, water, and carbon dioxide.

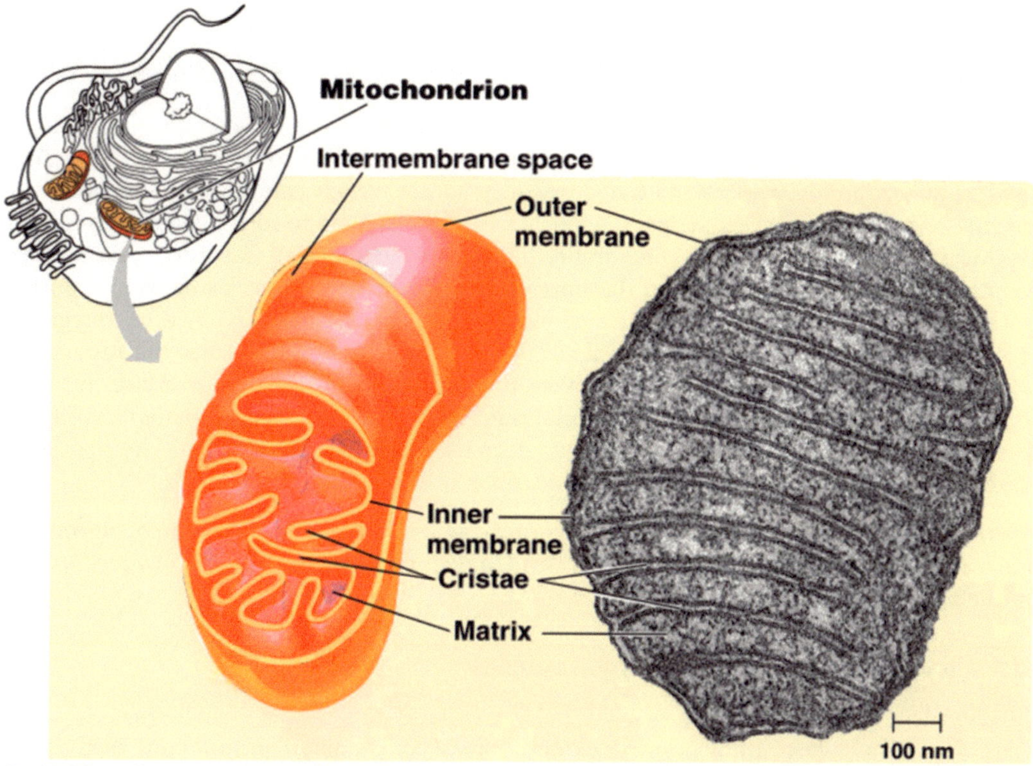

Fig. 2. Mitochondrial structure. (source: Pearson education, Inc., publishing as Benjamin Cummings).

1.2.2 Functions of mitochondria

One of the major mitochondrial functions is cellular respiration. It is a chemical process of releasing energy stored in glucose. The energy utilized in breaking down glucose is supplied by ATP molecules, and ATP molecules are produced by mitochondria. The entire process of aerobic cellular respiration is a three step process:

- Glycolysis: Glucose is a six carbon sugar. The enzymes in the cytoplasmic matrix initiate glycolysis in which a glucose molecule is oxidized to two molecules of three carbon sugars. Products of glycolysis are two molecules of ATP, two molecules of pyruvic acid and two NADH (Nicotinamide Adenine Dinucleotide) molecules (which are electron carrying molecules)

- Citric Acid Cycle (Krebs cycle): This is the second phase of cellular respiration. The three carbon molecules which have been produced as a result of glycolysis are converted into acetyl compounds. However, the intermediary reactions of this process yield ATP molecules of energy, NAD and FAD molecules too. NAD and FAD molecules are further reduced in the Citric Acid Cycle to high energy electrons
- Electron Transport: The electron transport chain is constituted of a series of electron carriers generated in the membrane of the mitochondria from Citric Acid Cycle. The ATP molecules are further produced by the chemical reactions of these electron carrier molecules. A eukaryotic cell produces about 36 ATP molecules after cellular respiration.

In fact, mitochondrial function in cellular energy metabolism is concerned with the processes of fatty acid and pyruvate oxidation, resulting in the formation of acetyl-CoA, which is subsequently oxidized in the Citric Acid Cycle. When combined, these processes generate reduced coenzymes, which deliver electrons to oxygen to form water, through the respiratory chain of the inner membrane. The whole process of fat and carbohydrate oxidation is strongly exergonic and the normal mitochondrion conserves the major part of this energy in the form of ADP phosphorylation to ATP. This dependence on oxygen is critical in skeletal muscle. Under normal circumstances, skeletal muscle has the capacity to increase its energy turnover, and this makes the transition from rest to exercise. Efficient oxygen delivery is very important for normal mitochondrial function, and patients suffering from peripheral arterial disease have a decreased blood flow to the legs due to arteriosclerosis, making less oxygen available to the mitochondria.

Other main mitochondrial functions are control of cell cycle, management of apoptosis, monitoring of cell differentiation, growth and development and reactive oxygen species production and clearance.

1.2.3 Mitochondria and reactive oxygen species

Mitochondria, main energy sources of the cells, are causes and targets of increased oxidative stress. Thus, the role of mitochondria extends far beyond energy production, as they are important generators of reactive oxygen species (ROS), which can act either as second messengers or as a source of cellular damage, depending on the produced amount. ROS are a double-edged sword: they are beneficial by playing an important role in cell signaling involved in antioxidant defense network, but could be harmful by inducing excessive oxidative stress resulting in protein carboxylation, lipids peroxydation and DNA damage. These free radicals have oxidizing properties, and they react in the environment where they are produced with a variety of biological substrates: fats, carbohydrates, proteins and DNA. There are also environmental factors that generate free radicals: pollution, sun exposure, smoking, consumption of alcohol or drugs, physical exercise. These situations induce an overproduction of reactive oxygen species. There are also defense systems that can regulate the production of theses species: free radicals are neutralized by enzymatic systems (superoxide dismutase, catalase and glutathione peroxidase), elements (copper, zinc, iron, selenium), as well as antioxidants such as vitamins A, C and E (Figure 3).

ROS include radical species such as primary superoxide $O_2^{\bullet-}$, and its conjugated acid hydroperoxyl radical $HO_2^{\bullet}$. Also included are the hydroxyl ($^{\bullet}OH$), carbonate ($CO_3^{\bullet -}$), peroxyl ($RO_2^{\bullet}$), and alkoxyl ($RO^{\bullet}$) radical. Also some non-radical species are ascribed to

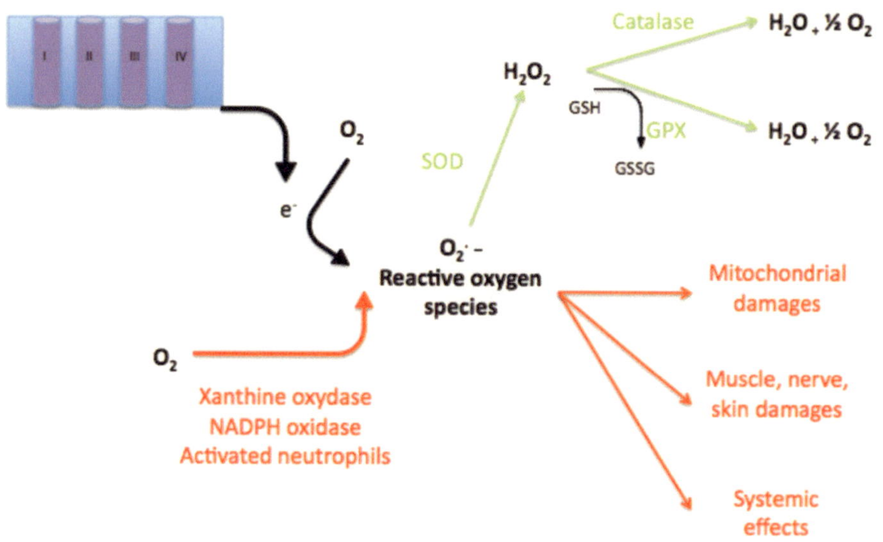

Fig. 3. Reactive oxygen species in peripheral arterial disease. SOD: superoxide dismutase; GPX: gluthatione peroxidase

ROS, namely H_2O_2, HOCl, fatty acid hydroperoxides (FAOOH), reactive aldehydes, singlet oxygen and other compounds (Chance *et al.*, 1979). Superoxide anion $O_2^{\bullet -}$ is the most important, it is a fairly stable compound, especially in an aqueous environment at neutral pH. Its toxicity is principally based on generation of further reactive species, called "downstream products" of $O_2^{\bullet -}$, which are then able to attack intracellular biomolecules.

There are currently seven separate sites of mitochondrial ROS production that have been identified (Figure 4) (Brand *et al.*, 2004).

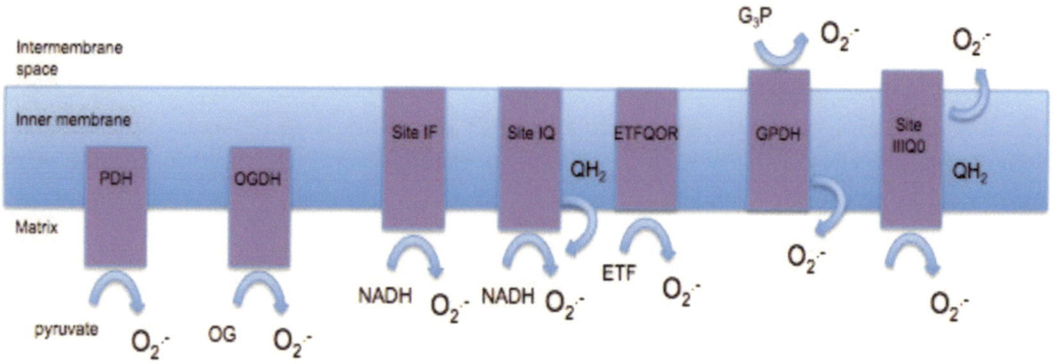

Fig. 4. Sites and topology of mitochondrial superoxide production. PDH: pyruvate dehydrogenase ; OGDH: 2-oxoglutarate dehydrogenase ; Site IF: NADH binding site of complex I ; Site IQ: uniquinine reduction site of complex I
ETFQOR: electron transferring flavoprotein ubiquinone oxidoreductase ; GPDH: glycerol 3-phosphate dehydrogenase
Site IIIQO: quinone binding site of the Q-cycle in complex III.

The relative importance of each site to total superoxide production in isolated mitochondria is contentious, partly because of different assays, different substrates and different sources of mitochondria. Most assays of superoxide production from defined sites measure maximal capacities for superoxide production, and the actual rate from each site in the absence of inhibitors is not known. During reverse electron transport from succinate to NAD+, complex I can produce superoxide at high rates (Han *et al.*, 2001; Votyakova & Reynolds, 2001; Kushnareva *et al.*, 2002; Liu *et al.*, 2002; Han *et al.*, 2003; Turrens, 2003; Lambert & Brand, 2004), although the physiological relevance is unclear (Votyakova & Reynolds, 2001). During forward electron transport from NAD-linked substrates (which may be more physiological), most mitochondria produce superoxide at high rates after addition of inhibitors such as rotenone (for complex I) (Han *et al.*, 2001; Liu *et al.*, 2002; St-Pierre *et al.*, 2002; Han *et al.*, 2003; Lambert & Brand, 2004) or antimycin A (for complex III)(Liu *et al.*, 2002; St-Pierre *et al.*, 2002; Muller *et al.*, 2004). Other physiologically relevant substrates, such as fatty acids and glycerol 3-phosphate, may cause superoxide production from sites that are less active during pyruvate oxidation, such as ETF-Q oxidoreductase and glycerol 3-phosphate dehydrogenase.

$O_2^{\bullet -}$ in the matrix is converted to H_2O_2 by matrix MnSOD, while $O_2^{\bullet -}$ released to the intramembrane space is partly dismuted by intermembrane space CuZnSOD (Inoue *et al.*, 2003). Any residual $O_2^{\bullet -}$ which diffuses into the cytosol is similarly converted by the cytosolic CuZnSOD. If any mitochondrial $O_2^{\bullet -}$ can reach the extracellular space, it is then detoxified by extracellular CuZnSOD (SOD_3) (Brand, 2010). Non-enzymatic lipoperoxidation is also a detoxification reaction. It can be considered not only as a detoxification reaction, but, due to its self-propagating nature, also as a new radical source initiated by the highly reactive radicals. Glutathione-based systems, including glutathione S transferase and the thioredoxin system, including peroxiredoxins, constitute the major redox buffer in the cytosol. Other detoxification systems (degrading H_2O_2 and ROS) are proteins of thioredoxin family, acting in concert with the thioredoxin-dependent peroxide reductase, and a family glutathione-S- transferase. H_2O_2 can be reduced to water by catalase or glutathione peroxidase, or alternatively to the hydroxyl radical in the presence of reduced copper or iron (Camello-Almaraz *et al.*, 2006).

Increased oxidative stress plays a key role in PAD and IR-induced muscular impairments. Both increased ROS secondary to mitochondrial dysfunction and decreased ROS catabolism are involved (Figures 1 and 3).

2. Mitochondrial and oxidative stress analysis of muscle biopsies

2.1 Histological methods

2.1.1 Histological analysis of skeletal muscle mitochondria

Mitochondria can be detected in confocal microscopy by conventional fluorescent stains, such as rhodamine 123 and tetramethylrosamine. These stains are readily sequestered by functioning mitochondria, but they are subsequently washed out of the cells once the mitochondrion's membrane potential is lost. This characteristic limits their use in experiments in which cells must be treated with aldehyde-based fixatives or other agents that affect the energetic state of the mitochondria. To overcome this limitation, it is possible to use a serie of mitochondrion selective stains (MitoTracker probes®) that are concentrated by active mitochondria and well retained during cell fixation. Because these mitochondrion selective stains are also retained following permeabilization, the sample retains the fluorescent staining pattern characteristic of live cells during subsequent processing steps for immunocytochemistry, in situ hybridization or electron microscopy.

MitoSOX® Red mitochondrial superoxide indicator is a fluorogenic dye for highly selective detection of superoxide in the mitochondria of live cells. It is live-cell permeant and is rapidly and selectively targeted to the mitochondria. Once in the mitochondria, it is oxidized by superoxide (but not by other reactive oxygen species) and exhibits red fluorescence. Oxidation of the probe is prevented by superoxide dismutase. The oxidation product becomes highly fluorescent (excitation/emission maxima of approximately 510/580 nm) upon binding to nucleic acids. Cells adhering to coverslips have to be covered by 1 or 2 mL of 5 μM of MitoSOX® reagent working solution, and incubated for 10 minutes at 37°C, protected from light. They are then washed gently three times with warm buffer, and mounted in warm buffer for confocal microscopy imaging (Mukhopadhyay *et al.*, 2007) (figure 5).

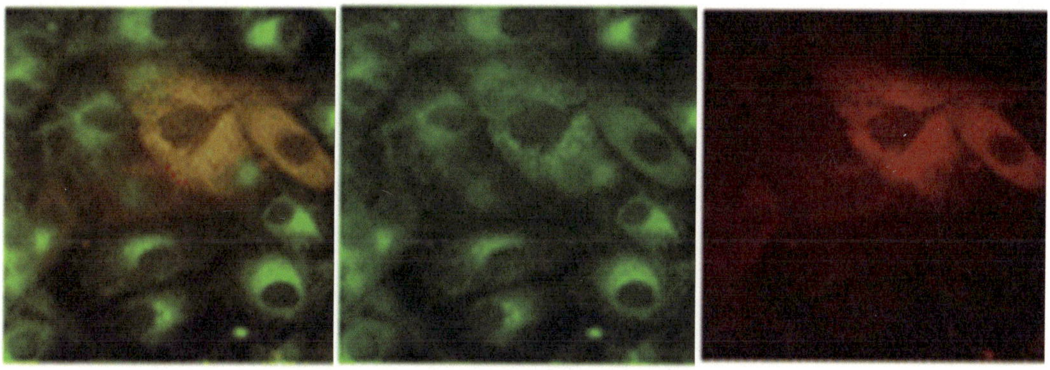

Merge MitoTracker MitoSOX

Fig. 5 Assessment of superoxide generation. MitoSOX Red stain (top panel) revealed the presence of superoxide anion MitoSOX Red colocalized with MitoTracker Green (middle panel) in merged images (bottom panels), indicating that the excess superoxide anion was concentrated in mitochondria (Quinzii *et al.*, 2008).

In transmission electron microscopy, mitochondrial ultrastructure can be studied. The material is fixed, embedded, sectioned, and then examined. It is important to note that the sections must be less than 0.1 μm in thickness, even less than 0.05 μm, in order to show the structural details described with enough clarity for profitable study of the mitochondria (Frey *et al.*, 2002) (figure 6).

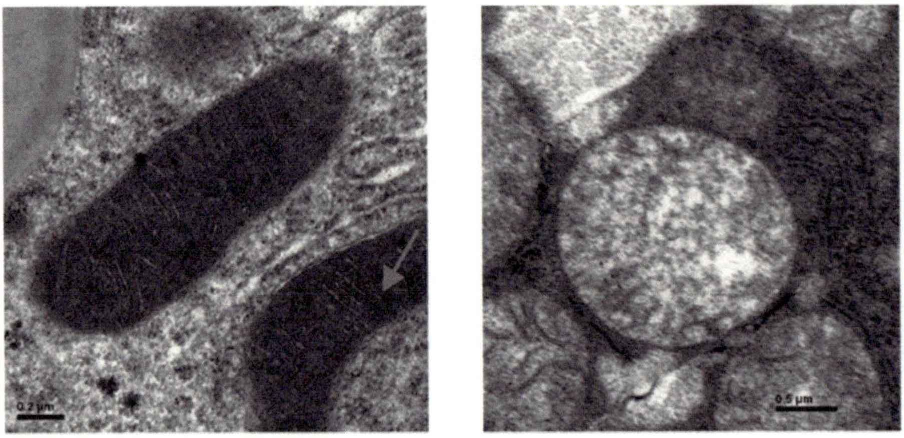

Fig. 6. Micrographs of transmission electron microscopy sections of mitochondria, TEM ×60K. The left photo represent a healthy mitochondrion the arrow indicates the cristae; the right photo represents a swelling mitochondrion (Li *et al.*, 2010).

2.1.2 Microscopy fluorescence: Dihydroethidium staining

To detect the presence of ROS in skeletal muscles, serial sections (10 µm-thick) are cut on a cryostat microtome, mounted into glass slides and incubated with 2.5 µM dihydroethidium (DHE). DHE produces red fluorescence when oxidized to ethidium bromide (EtBr), mainly by superoxide anion. After staining, sections are examined under an epifluorescence microscope (Nikon Eclipse E800) and emission signal are recorded with a Zeiss filter (Dikalov *et al.*, 2007) (figure 7).

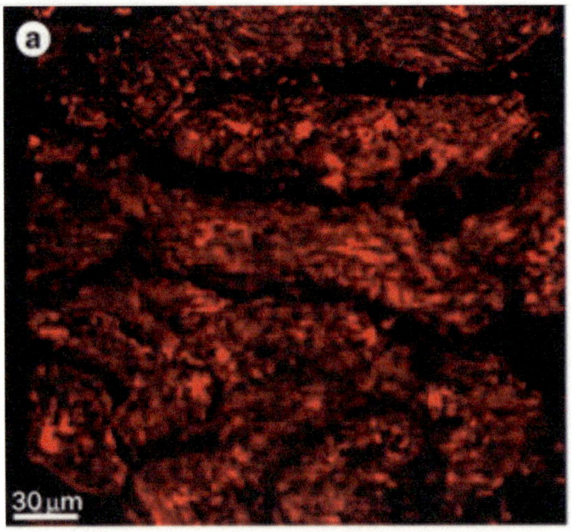

Fig. 7. A representative photo of Superoxide production by dihydroethidium staining of tissue in the acute phase of stress cardiomyopathy (Nef et al., 2008)

Inhibitors of NADPH oxidase (diphenylene iodonium) and xanthine oxidase are known to reduce mitochondrial superoxide production through inhibiting NADH ubiquinone oxidoreductase (complex I) (Riganti *et al.*, 2004).

2.2 Functional methods

2.2.1 Mitochondrial respiratory chain complexes activities using saponin skinned fibres

The mitochondrial respiratory chain complexes activities study is described in an other chapter. This technique is based on the measure of oxygen consumption in skinned fibres in order to determine the functional oxidative capacity of the skeletal muscle in its cellular environment (Veksler *et al.*, 1987; Riganti *et al.*, 2004) (see the chapter from Charles et al. for much more explanations and the description of the methods).

2.2.2 H_2O_2 Production in permeabilized fibres

H_2O_2 production is assessed in permeabilized fibres (Kuznetsov *et al.*, 2008) in response to sequential addition of substrates and inhibitors (Anderson & Neufer, 2006). H_2O_2 production is measured with Amplex Red reagent (Invitrogen), which reacts with H_2O_2 in a 1:1 stoichiometry catalyzed by HRP (Horse Radish Peroxidase; Fluka Biochemika) to yield the fluorescent compound resorufin and molar equivalent O2. Resorufin has excitation/emission characteristics of 563/587 nm and is extremely stable once formed. Fluorescence is measured continuously [change in fluorescence (ΔF)/sec] with a spectrofluorometer with temperature control and magnetic stirring. After a baseline, ΔF (reactants only) is established; the reaction is initiated by addition of a permeabilized fibre bundle to 600 µl of buffer Z with glutamate (5µM) and malate (2.5µM) as substrates for complex I and succinate (5mM) for complex II. ADP (2mM) is injected in the reaction buffer and led to a reduction in H_2O_2 release, which is expected when electron flow through the respiratory chain is stimulated. Finally, addition of the complex I inhibitor amytal (2mM) and the complex III inhibitor antimycin (8µM) led to interruption of normal electron flow and induced an increase in H_2O_2 release.

3. Mitochondrial dysfunctions during peripheral arterial disease

During PAD, significant muscles ischemia/reperfusion is well known to induce skeletal muscles alterations (Figure 1). The pathogenesis of PAD manifestations is lead to the development of athero-occlusive disease in the lower limb arteries. Arterial stenoses usually do not affect the blood supply at rest, but at the time of walking or other exercise, they make the leg ischemic and painful forcing the patient to rest. At rest, perfusion returns again to normal levels. These cycles of ischemia and reperfusion launch a cascade of inflammatory changes and induce the production of ROS in the skeletal muscle. Multiple daily ischemia/reperfusion events initiated by simple activities such as walking result, over time, in morphological and ultrastructural changes in both the contractile element of the muscle and its mitochondria. Dysfunctional mitochondria then further lower the already decreased (by compromised blood supply) energy levels in the pathologic muscle and become sources of ever increasing levels of ROS and possibly inducers of apoptosis. A vicious cycle is thus initiated gradually leading to deteriorating mitochondrial function and escalating ROS production with ongoing damage of every structure in the myocytes. Apoptosis, along with cellular necrosis (from ischemia, reactive oxygen species, and low energy levels), may then be induced, eventually leading to a severe myopathy that significantly affects the function and performance of PAD limbs. In addition, nerves, skin, and subcutaneous tissues damages are formed, ultimately leading to the characteristically atrophic legs of patients with advanced PAD having thin muscles; brittle, hairless, and thin skin with shiny texture; and impaired sensorimotor function. On the basis of these concepts, it is easy to understand how claudication, rest pain, and tissue loss find their place in the heart of this continuum of events, coming into view as the external manifestations of ongoing tissue injury and deterioration (Blaisdell, 2002; Pipinos *et al.*, 2008a).

3.1 Selected experimental data (Table 1)

Author	Journal	Year	Histology	Oxidative stress	Respirometry
Makris	Vascular	2007	Myopathic features Drop in total protein content Increased mitochondrial content	Increased oxidative stress	Bioenergetic decline Inadequate oxidative phosphorylation Decreased ATP energy production
Pipinos II	J Vasc Surg	2000	Myopathic features Increased mitochondrial content, more oxidative type fibres.	- Increased oxidative stress : xanthine oxidase and activated neutrophils are source of ROS - Alteration of activity and expression of MnSOD. - Damage to mtDNA	Decreased activities of complexes I, III, and IV.
Pipinos II	Vasc Endovasc Surg	2008b			
Brass	Vasc Med	1996 2000			
Wallace	Am Heart J	2000	Increased mitochondrial content	Increased oxidative stress	-
Levak-Frank	J Clin Invest	1996	Increased mitochondrial content	-	-
Wredenberg	Proc Nath Acad Sci USA	1999			

Table 1. Experimental data

Peripheral arterial disease is a consequence of compromised blood supply to the ischemic limb (Brass, 1996; Brass & Hiatt, 2000). Experimental data show that skeletal muscle responds to inflow arterial occlusion with the development of myopathic histological changes, a drop in total protein content, and a trend toward decreased wet weight (Makris, et al., 2007 ; Pipinos, et al., 2008b). Peripheral arterial disease is characterized by a significant increase in the mitochondrial content of skeletal muscle, and mitochondrial proliferation is characteristic of mitochondrial diseases and aging (Levak-Frank *et al.*, 1995; Wallace, 2000; Wredenberg *et al.*, 2002; Makris *et al.*, 2007; Pipinos *et al.*, 2008b). In skeletal muscle, an upregulation of mitochondrial biogenesis may be associated with and alteration of muscle fibre type toward the more oxidative type I and IIa fibres (Pipinos *et al.*, 2008b).

Defective mitochondria are central to this myopathy, through compromised performance as primary energy producers and regulators of oxygen radical species. Thus, PAD myopathy is characterized by an increased content of dysfunctional mitochondria having significant defects in electron transport chain complexes I, III, and IV (Pipinos *et al.*, 2000; Pipinos *et al.*, 2008b). These defects are associated with a bioenergetic decline, characterized by inadequate oxidative phosphorylation, decreased ATP energy production, and increased oxidative stress (Makris *et al.*, 2007; Pipinos *et al.*, 2008b). Ischemic skeletal muscle sustains substantial oxidative injuries indicated by an increase in protein carbonylation and lipid peroxidation adducts. Under resting conditions, a large proportion of cellular reactive oxygen species is produced in the mitochondria (Wallace, 2000).

Thus, ischemia/reperfusion is the central problem in animals with inflow arterial occlusion (Brevetti *et al.*, 2001). Ischemia/reperfusion increases oxidative stress, triggers inflammation and oxidative damage to the tissues, and initiates mitochondrial injury and dysfunction. Mitochondrial dysfunction can then be perpetuated by repeated destructive cycles of ischemia/reperfusion, causing amplification of respiratory chain defects, compromised bioenergetics, increased reactive oxygen species production, diminished MnSOD antioxidant activity. The combination of compromised bioenergetics and worsening oxidative stress may then lead to progressive oxidative damage of structures in the myocytes (Brass, 1996; Brass & Hiatt, 2000; Makris *et al.*, 2007; Pipinos *et al.*, 2008a).

There are non-invasive techniques that can evaluate *in vivo* the mitochondrial energy transformation by the monitoring of the tissue oxygen level: either directly with the ^{31}phosphorous magnetic resonance spectroscopy (Hands *et al.*, 1990; Greiner *et al.*, 2006), or indirectly with infrared spectroscopy (Hands *et al.*, 1986; Watanabe *et al.*, 2004; Ubbink & Koopman, 2006). The ^{31}phosphorous magnetic resonance spectroscopy is used to determine the concentrations of metabolites involved in muscle energy metabolism (phosphocreatin, inorganic phosphate, and ATP). From these data, free ADP and pH may be calculated (Quistorff *et al.*, 1993). The infrared spectroscopy is used to measure the state of oxygen saturation in hemoglobin and myoglobin in blood and muscle at a given time and a given location. It can be considered as an indirect measure of the muscle perfusion versus oxygen consumption (Comerota *et al.*, 2003).

Mitochondrial function may also be evaluated by respirometry on muscle biopsies. The feasibility, indications, contra-indications are now well known and such a technique become usual in specialized centers. Thus, skeletal muscle biopsies can be obtained during surgery, or they can be obtained under local anesthesia. Biopsy sites can be anesthetized with a 2%

lidocaine solution, and 1.0 cm incisions can be made through the skin and gastrocnemius fascia. A modified 5 mm Bergstrom biopsy needle can then be inserted 10-15 mm and used to obtain 40 to 50 mg of skeletal muscle. Contraindications are essentially represented by bleeding disorders, infection at biopsy sites, or allergy to local anesthetics.

3.2 Selected clinical data (Table 2)

<table>
<tr><th>Author</th><th>Journal</th><th>Year</th><th>Histology</th><th>Oxidative stress</th><th>Respirometry</th></tr>
<tr><td>Makris</td><td>Vascular</td><td>2007</td><td rowspan="4">Myopathic features

Increased mitochondrial content

More type I fibres</td><td>Increased oxidative stress</td><td>Bioenergetic decline</td></tr>
<tr><td>Pipinos II</td><td>J Vasc Surg</td><td>2000</td><td rowspan="2">Increased oxidative stress : xanthine oxidase and activated neutrophils are source of ROS

Alteration of activity and expression of MnSOD

Damage to mtDNA</td><td rowspan="3">Decreased activities of complexes I, III, and IV.</td></tr>
<tr><td>Pipinos II</td><td>Vasc Endovasc Surg</td><td>2008</td></tr>
<tr><td>Brass</td><td>Vasc Med</td><td>2000</td><td>Increased oxidative stress</td></tr>
</table>

Table 2. Clinical data.

Previous studies have shown that PAD is associated with alterations in skeletal muscle histology (Brass & Hiatt, 2000; Makris *et al.*, 2007; Pipinos *et al.*, 2008b). Necrotic and regenerating fibres as well as inflammation have been seen in the diseased legs in comparison to contralateral legs of patients with unilateral peripheral arterial disease hospitalized for surgical evaluation. Furthermore, in the setting of aortic aneurysm repair in human, light microscopy revealed a consistent granulocyte infiltration in the ischemic and reperfused skeletal muscle. Ultrastructural damage to the muscle fibers was seen during ischemia and became more severe upon reperfusion. The recruitment of granulocytes into the muscle tissue paralleled the activation of the blood complement system and an increase in circulating neutrophils (Formigli L *et al.*, 1992).

3.2.1 Patients with functional ischemia

The 31phosphorous magnetic resonance spectroscopy examination shows a higher inorganic phosphate/phosphocreatin ratio compared to control patients (Hands *et al.*, 1986; Zatina *et al.*, 1986; Hands *et al.*, 1990). The infrared spectroscopy examination shows a large drop in the oxygen saturation in the muscle and an increased oxygenation recovery time after exercise when compared to control patients (Kemp *et al.*, 2001; Comerota *et al.*, 2003). Histological examination shows more type I muscle fibres containing a high amount of mitochondria in the gastrocnemius muscle of patients with functional ischemia. In addition, the severity of the peripheral arterial disease was correlated with the increased percentage of type I fibres (Makitie & Teravainen, 1977).

3.2.2 Patients with critical limb ischemia

The 31phosphorous magnetic resonance spectroscopy examination shows a higher intracellular pH, and a higher inorganic phosphate/phosphocreatin ratio compared to control patients (Hands *et al.*, 1986; Zatina *et al.*, 1986; Hands *et al.*, 1990). The infrared spectroscopy examination shows a large decrease in the oxygen saturation in the muscle and an increased oxygenation recovery after surgery. Respirometry shows a reduced mitochondrial respiratory rate in the gastrocnemius muscle compared to control patients (Pipinos *et al.*, 2003; Pipinos *et al.*, 2006). The reduced respiratory rate is specifically located to complexes I, III and IV enzymes of the respiratory chain; probably due to reactive oxygen species generated damage (Sjostrom *et al.*, 1980; Pipinos *et al.*, 2003).

4. Improving mitochondrial function and reducing oxidative stress: selected experimental and clinical results (Table 3)

Author	Journal	Year	Type	Histology	Oxidative stress	Respiro-metry	Necrosis
Tran	Eur J Pharmacol	2011	Pre	-	Decreased superoxide production	C I, III and IV activities normalized	Reduced infarct size
Andreadou	Mini Rev Med Chem	2008a,b	Pre Post	-	-	-	
Martou	J Appli Physiol	2006	Pre	Normal morphology	-	-	-
Addison	Am J Physiol Heart Circ Physiol	2003	Pre	Attenuation of neutrophil accumulation	Decreased oxidative stress	No bioenergetic decline	-
Thaveau	J Vasc Surg	2007	Pre	-	-	Restoration of complexes I and II activities	-

Okorie	Eur Heart J	2011	Post	-	Decreased oxidative stress by inihibition of the opening of mPTP	-	-
McAllister	Am J Physiol Regul Integr Comp Physiol	2008	Post				
Eberlin	Plast Reconstr Surg	2009	Post	Decreased of injured fibres	-	-	Reduced infarct size
Charles	Br J Surg	2011	Post	-	Decreased oxidative stress Preserved antioxydant defense	Increased complexes I, II, III, and IV activities	-
Tsubota	Eur J Vasc Endovasc Surg	2010	Post	Attenuation of neutrophil accumulation	-	-	Reduced tissue necrosis

Table 3. Effects of pre- and post-conditioning. This table summarizes clinical studies realized on pre- or postconditioning.

4.1 Ischemic pre- and post-conditioning

Besides reducing preoperative ischemic time and surgery duration, ischemic preconditioning -defined as brief episodes of ischemia/reperfusion applied before sustained ischemia- decreases skeletal muscle mitochondrial dysfunction, enhances limb and remotes organ protections. Furthermore, remote and local ischemic preconditioning equivalently protects skeletal muscle mitochondrial function during experimental aortic cross-clamping (Mansour *et al.*, in Press). Nevertheless, ischemia occurrence is difficult to predict and might limit a broader use of ischemic preconditioning. Controlled reperfusion appears thus as a valuable therapeutic approach after limb ischemia and ischemic post-conditioning, characterized by repeated cycles of IR performed at the onset of reperfusion, appeared safe and easy to perform.

Ischemic preconditioning has been mainly elucidated in experimental cardiac ischemia. Ischemic preconditioning utilizes endogenous as well as distant mechanisms in skeletal muscle, liver, lung, kidney, intestine and brain in animal models to convey varying degrees of protection from ischemia/reperfusion injury (Ambros *et al.*, 2007). Specifically, preconditioned tissues exhibit altered energy metabolism, better electrolyte homeostasis and genetic reorganization, as well as less oxygen-free radicals and activated neutrophils release, reduced apoptosis and better microcirculatory perfusion. To date, there are few human studies, but trials suggest that different organ in human such as heart, liver, lung and skeletal muscle acquire protection after ischemia/reperfusion (Sjostrom *et al.*, 1980; Ali *et al.*,2007; Cheung M *et al.*, 1996; Kharbanda *et al.*, 2002). It has been showed that ischemic preconditioning positively influenced muscle metabolism during reperfusion, and this, results in an increase in phosphocreatin production and higher oxygen consumption (Andreas *et al.*, 2011).

Experimental data showed that ischemic postconditioning confers protection against different organ injuries caused by longer circulatory occlusions during elective major vascular surgeries, because it causes a significant reduction in systemic inflammatory response (TNF-alpha, oxygen-derived free radicals) (Eberlin *et al.*, 2009). Besides the heart (Skyschally *et al.*,2009), postconditioning is also effective in salvage of ischemic skeletal muscle from reperfusion injury and the mechanism likely involves inhibition of opening of the mPTP and/or reduced oxidative stress (Szijarto *et al.*,2009; Tsubota *et al.*, 2010; Park *et al.*, 2010; Guyrkovic *et al.*, 2011; Mc Allister *et al.*, 2008; Charles *et al.*, 2011). There are few human studies, but it has been showed that postconditioning by intermittent early reperfusion reduces ischemia/reperfusion injury, that might depend on K(ATP) channel activation, and is mimicked by inhibition of the mPTP at reperfusion (Okorie *et al.*, 2011).

4.2 Pharmacological protection of skeletal muscle in the setting of ischemia/reperfusion

Although preconditioning is a powerful form of protection, its clinical application is limited because of practical reasons. In fact, the short ischemic insults in preconditioning have to be applied before the onset of sustained period of ischemia which cannot be precisely anticipated. On the contrary, the very brief insults in postconditioning have to be applied immediately after the end of the long ischemia thus making the intervention more easily applicable. Both mechanisms limit the reperfusion injury but easier approaches deserve to be studied.

Pharmacological preconditioning and postconditioning represent ideal alternatives that may substitute the short ischemic insults for pharmaceuticals means. The components of preconditioning share two main pathways, one that involves the mitochondrial K(ATP) channels- free radicals and PKC and another one that involves adenosine and PKC. Reperfusion injury salvage kinases (RISK) prevent the mitochondrial permeability transition pores (mPTP) opening which destroy the mitochondria and cause cell death. PC *via* PKC and postconditioning *via* gradual restoration of pH at reperfusion up-regulate RISK and preserve viable part of the ischemic region. In order to confer pharmacological protection, novel therapeutic strategies, based on the knowledge of the ligands, of the receptors and of the intracellular signaling pathways have emerged (Addison *et al.*, 2003; Gamboa *et al.*, 2003; Martou *et al.*, 2006; Andreadou *et al.*, 2008b). Adenosine, nicorandil, tempol, coenzyme Q and other agents (Addison *et al.*, 2003; Gamboa *et al.*, 2003; Martou *et al.*, 2006; Thaveau *et al.*, 2010) have been already used as pharmacological mimetics of ischemic preconditioning. Furthermore, agents that increase RISK or directly prevent mPTP are also under investigation as postconditioning analogues (Andreadou *et al.*, 2008a; Tsubota *et al.*, 2010; Tran *et al.*, 2011). Antioxidant systems are also important: several endogenous antioxidant systems are found in muscle tissue, these include alpha-tocopherol, histidine-containing dipeptides, and antioxidant enzymes such as glutathione peroxidase, superoxide dismutase, and catalase. The contribution of alpha-tocopherol to the oxidative stability of skeletal muscle is largely influenced by diet. Dietary supplementation of tocopherol has been shown to increase muscle alpha-tocopherol concentrations and to inhibit lipid oxidation. Dietary selenium supplementation has also been shown to increase the oxidative stability of muscle presumably by increasing the activity of glutathione peroxidase, and dietary restriction improves systemic and muscular oxidative stress (Rodrigues *et al.*, 2011). The oxidative stability of skeletal muscle is also influenced by the histidine-containing dipeptides, carnosine and anserine (Chan & Decker, 1994).

5. Conclusions / Perspectives

Mitochondria are the main energy source of the cells and mitochondrial dysfunction is associated with cell and organ impairment. Consistently, IR has been shown to induce skeletal muscle mitochondrial dysfunctions in animals and humans and improving skeletal muscle mitochondrial function is an interesting and clinically pertinent therapeutic goal. Indeed, improving skeletal muscle mitochondrial function enhances walking capacities in patients suffering from peripheral arterial disease.

Muscle biopsy allows to precisely determine the deleterious effects of IR on skeletal muscle and can be used to better stratify patient's risk and to guide therapy. Ischemic pre- and post-conditioning and pharmacologic conditioning allows protection of skeletal muscle in the setting of ischemia/reperfusion, decreasing mitochondrial respiratory chain injury, reducing reactive oxygen species (ROS) production and enhancing muscles antioxidant defence.

Future work will be useful to determine whether even smaller biopsies, analyzed after being frozen, might yield the same information.

6. References

Addison PD, Neligan PC, Ashrafpour H, Khan A, Zhong A, Moses M, Forrest CR & Pang CY. (2003). Noninvasive remote ischemic preconditioning for global protection of skeletal muscle against infarction. *Am J Physiol Heart Circ Physiol* 285, H1435-1443.

Ali ZA, Callaghan CJ, Lim E, Ali AA, Nouraei SA, Akthar AM, Boyle JR, Varty K, Kharbanda RK, Dutka DP, & Gaunt ME. (2007). Remote ischemic preconditioning reduces myocardial and renal injury after elective abdominal aortic aneurysm repair: a randomized controlled trial. *Circulation* 116,I98-105.

Ambros JT, Herrero-Fresneda I, Borau OG & Boira JM. (2007). Ischemic preconditioning in solid organ transplantation: from experimental to clinics. *Transpl Int* 20, 219-229.

Anderson EJ & Neufer PD. (2006). Type II skeletal myofibers possess unique properties that potentiate mitochondrial H(2)O(2) generation. *Am J Physiol Cell Physiol* 290, C844-851.

Andreadou I, Iliodromitis EK, Koufaki M, Farmakis D, Tsotinis A & Kremastinos DT. (2008a). Alternative pharmacological interventions that limit myocardial infarction. *Curr Med Chem* 15, 3204-3213.

Andreadou I, Iliodromitis EK, Koufaki M & Kremastinos DT. (2008b). Pharmacological pre- and post- conditioning agents: reperfusion-injury of the heart revisited. *Mini Rev Med Chem* 8, 952-959.

Andreas M, Schmid AI, Keilani M, Doberer D, Bartko J, Crevenna R, Moser E & Wolzt M. (2011). Effect of ischemic preconditioning in skeletal muscle measured by functional magnetic resonance imaging and spectroscopy: a randomized crossover trial. *J Cardiovasc Magn Reson* 13, 32.

Bhat HK, Hiatt WR, Hoppel CL & Brass EP. (1999). Skeletal muscle mitochondrial DNA injury in patients with unilateral peripheral arterial disease. *Circulation* 99, 807-812.

Blaisdell FW. (2002). The pathophysiology of skeletal muscle ischemia and the reperfusion syndrome: a review. *Cardiovasc Surg* 10, 620-630.

Brand MD. (2010). The sites and topology of mitochondrial superoxide production. *Exp Gerontol* 45, 466-472.

Brand MD, Affourtit C, Esteves TC, Green K, Lambert AJ, Miwa S, Pakay JL & Parker N. (2004). Mitochondrial superoxide: production, biological effects, and activation of uncoupling proteins. *Free Radic Biol Med* 37, 755-767.

Brass EP. (1996). Skeletal muscle metabolism as a target for drug therapy in peripheral arterial disease. *Vasc Med* 1, 55-59.

Brass EP & Hiatt WR. (2000). Acquired skeletal muscle metabolic myopathy in atherosclerotic peripheral arterial disease. *Vasc Med* 5, 55-59.

Brass EP, Hiatt WR, Gardner AW & Hoppel CL. (2001). Decreased NADH dehydrogenase and ubiquinol-cytochrome c oxidoreductase in peripheral arterial disease. *Am J Physiol Heart Circ Physiol* 280, H603-609.

Brevetti LS, Paek R, Brady SE, Hoffman JI, Sarkar R & Messina LM. (2001). Exercise-induced hyperemia unmasks regional blood flow deficit in experimental hindlimb ischemia. *J Surg Res* 98, 21-26.

Camello-Almaraz C, Gomez-Pinilla PJ, Pozo MJ & Camello PJ. (2006). Mitochondrial reactive oxygen species and Ca2+ signaling. *Am J Physiol Cell Physiol* 291, C1082-1088.

Chan KM & Decker EA. (1994). Endogenous skeletal muscle antioxidants. *Crit Rev Food Sci Nutr* 34, 403-426.

Chance B, Sies H & Boveris A. (1979). Hydroperoxide metabolism in mammalian organs. *Physiol Rev* 59, 527-605.

Charles AL, Guilbert AS, Bouitbir J, Goette-Di Marco P, Enache I, Zoll J, Piquard F & Geny B. (2011). Effect of postconditioning on mitochondrial dysfunction in experimental aortic cross-clamping. *Br J Surg* 98, 511-516.

Cheung MM, Kharbanda RK & Konstantinov IE. (2006). Randomized controlled trial of the effects of the remote ischemix preconditioning on children undergoing cardiac surgery: first clinical application in humans. *J Am Coll Cardiol* 47, 2277-2282.

Comerota AJ, Throm RC, Kelly P & Jaff M. (2003). Tissue (muscle) oxygen saturation (StO2): a new measure of symptomatic lower-extremity arterial disease. *J Vasc Surg* 38, 724-729.

Dikalov S, Griendling KK & Harrison DG. (2007). Measurement of reactive oxygen species in cardiovascular studies. *Hypertension* 49, 717-727.

Eberlin KR, McCormack MC, Nguyen JT, Tatlidede HS, Randolph MA & Austen WG, Jr. (2009). Sequential limb ischemia demonstrates remote postconditioning protection of murine skeletal muscle. *Plast Reconstr Surg* 123, 8S-16S.

Fontaine R, Kim M & Kieny R. (1954). [Surgical treatment of peripheral circulation disorders]. *Helv Chir Acta* 21, 499-533.

Formigli L, Lombardo LD, Adembri C, Brunelleschi S, Ferrari E, Novelli GP. Neutrophils as mediators to human skeletal muscle ischemia-reperfusion syndrome. Hum Pathol 1992;23:627-34.

Frey TG, Renken CW & Perkins GA. (2002). Insight into mitochondrial structure and function from electron tomography. *Biochim Biophys Acta* 1555, 196-203.

Gamboa A, Ertl AC, Costa F, Farley G, Manier ML, Hachey DL, Diedrich A & Biaggioni I. (2003). Blockade of nucleoside transport is required for delivery of intraarterial adenosine into the interstitium: relevance to therapeutic preconditioning in humans. *Circulation* 108, 2631-2635.

Greiner A, Esterhammer R, Messner H, Biebl M, Muhlthaler H, Fraedrich G, Jaschke WR & Schocke MF. (2006). High-energy phosphate metabolism during incremental calf exercise in patients with unilaterally symptomatic peripheral arterial disease measured by phosphor 31 magnetic resonance spectroscopy. *J Vasc Surg* 43, 978-986.

Gyurkovics E, Aranyi P, Stangl R, Onody P, Ferreira G, Lotz G, Kupcsulik P, & Szijarto A. (2011). Postconditioning of the lower limb - protection against the reperfusion syndrome. *J Surg Res* 169,139-147.

Han D, Antunes F, Canali R, Rettori D & Cadenas E. (2003). Voltage-dependent anion channels control the release of the superoxide anion from mitochondria to cytosol. *J Biol Chem* 278, 5557-5563.

Han D, Williams E & Cadenas E. (2001). Mitochondrial respiratory chain-dependent generation of superoxide anion and its release into the intermembrane space. *Biochem J* 353, 411-416.

Hands LJ, Payne GS, Bore PJ, Morris PJ & Radda GK. (1986). Magnetic resonance spectroscopy in ischaemic feet. *Lancet* 2, 1391.

Hands LJ, Sharif MH, Payne GS, Morris PJ & Radda GK. (1990). Muscle ischaemia in peripheral vascular disease studied by 31P-magnetic resonance spectroscopy. *Eur J Vasc Surg* 4, 637-642.

Inoue M, Sato EF, Nishikawa M, Park AM, Kira Y, Imada I & Utsumi K. (2003). Mitochondrial generation of reactive oxygen species and its role in aerobic life. *Curr Med Chem* 10, 2495-2505.

Kemp GJ, Roberts N, Bimson WE, Bakran A, Harris PL, Gilling-Smith GL, Brennan J, Rankin A & Frostick SP. (2001). Mitochondrial function and oxygen supply in normal and in chronically ischemic muscle: a combined 31P magnetic resonance spectroscopy and near infrared spectroscopy study in vivo. *J Vasc Surg* 34, 1103-1110.

Kharbanda RK, Motensen UM, White PA, Kristiansen SB, Schmidt MR, Hoschtitsky JA, Vogel M, Sorensen K, Redington AN, & MacAllister R. (2002). Transient lim ischemia induces remote ischemic preconditioning in vivo. *Circulation* 106,2881-2883.

Kushnareva Y, Murphy AN & Andreyev A. (2002). Complex I-mediated reactive oxygen species generation: modulation by cytochrome c and NAD(P)+ oxidation-reduction state. *Biochem J* 368, 545-553.

Kuznetsov AV, Veksler V, Gellerich FN, Saks V, Margreiter R & Kunz WS. (2008). Analysis of mitochondrial function in situ in permeabilized muscle fibers, tissues and cells. *Nat Protoc* 3, 965-976.

Lambert AJ & Brand MD. (2004). Inhibitors of the quinone-binding site allow rapid superoxide production from mitochondrial NADH:ubiquinone oxidoreductase (complex I). *J Biol Chem* 279, 39414-39420.

Levak-Frank S, Radner H, Walsh A, Stollberger R, Knipping G, Hoefler G, Sattler W, Weinstock PH, Breslow JL & Zechner R. (1995). Muscle-specific overexpression of lipoprotein lipase causes a severe myopathy characterized by proliferation of mitochondria and peroxisomes in transgenic mice. *J Clin Invest* 96, 976-986.

Li YG, Ji DF, Zhong S, Shi LG, Hu GY & Chen S. (2010). Saponins from Panax japonicus protect against alcohol-induced hepatic injury in mice by up-regulating the expression of GPX3, SOD1 and SOD3. *Alcohol Alcohol* 45, 320-331.

Liu Y, Fiskum G & Schubert D. (2002). Generation of reactive oxygen species by the mitochondrial electron transport chain. *J Neurochem* 80, 780-787.

Lundgren F, Dahllof AG, Schersten T & Bylund-Fellenius AC. (1989). Muscle enzyme adaptation in patients with peripheral arterial insufficiency: spontaneous adaptation, effect of different treatments and consequences on walking performance. *Clin Sci (Lond)* 77, 485-493.

Makitie J & Teravainen H. (1977). Histochemical changes in striated muscle in patients with intermittent claudication. *Arch Pathol Lab Med* 101, 658-663.

Makris KI, Nella AA, Zhu Z, Swanson SA, Casale GP, Gutti TL, Judge AR & Pipinos, II. (2007). Mitochondriopathy of peripheral arterial disease. *Vascular* 15, 336-343.

Mansour Z, Bouitbir J, Charles AL, Talha S, Kindo M, Pottecher J, Zoll J & Geny B. (in Press). Remote and local ischemic preconditioning equivatently protects rats skeletal muscle mitochondrial function during experimental aortic cross-clamping. *J Vasc Surg.*

Marbini A, Gemignani F, Scoditti U, Rustichelli P, Bragaglia MM & Govoni E. (1986). Abnormal muscle mitochondria in ischemic claudication. *Acta Neurol Belg* 86, 304-310.

Martou G, O'Blenes CA, Huang N, McAllister SE, Neligan PC, Ashrafpour H, Pang CY & Lipa JE. (2006). Development of an in vitro model for study of the efficacy of ischemic preconditioning in human skeletal muscle against ischemia-reperfusion injury. *J Appl Physiol* 101, 1335-1342.

McAllister SE, Ashrafpour H, Cahoon N, Huang N, Moses MA, Neligan PC, Forrest CR, Lipa JE & Pang CY. (2008). Postconditioning for salvage of ischemic skeletal muscle from reperfusion injury: efficacy and mechanism. *Am J Physiol Regul Integr Comp Physiol* 295, R681-689.

Mukhopadhyay P, Rajesh M, Yoshihiro K, Hasko G & Pacher P. (2007). Simple quantitative detection of mitochondrial superoxide production in live cells. *Biochem Biophys Res Commun* 358, 203-208.

Muller FL, Liu Y & Van Remmen H. (2004). Complex III releases superoxide to both sides of the inner mitochondrial membrane. *J Biol Chem* 279, 49064-49073.

Nef HM, Mollmann H, Troidl C, Kostin S, Bottger T, Voss S, Hilpert P, Krause N, Weber M, Rolf A, Dill T, Schaper J, Hamm CW & Elsasser A. (2008). Expression profiling of cardiac genes in Tako-Tsubo cardiomyopathy: insight into a new cardiac entity. *J Mol Cell Cardiol* 44, 395-404.

Norgren L, Hiatt WR, Dormandy JA, Nehler MR, Harris KA, Fowkes FG, Bell K, Caporusso J, Durand-Zaleski I, Komori K, Lammer J, Liapis C, Novo S, Razavi M, Robbs J, Schaper N, Shigematsu H, Sapoval M, White C, White J, Clement D, Creager M, Jaff M, Mohler E, 3rd, Rutherford RB, Sheehan P, Sillesen H & Rosenfield K. (2007). Inter-Society Consensus for the Management of Peripheral Arterial Disease (TASC II). *Eur J Vasc Endovasc Surg* 33 Suppl 1, S1-75.

Okorie MI, Bhavsar DD, Ridout D, Charakida M, Deanfield JE, Loukogeorgakis SP & MacAllister RJ. (2011). Postconditioning protects against human endothelial ischaemia-reperfusion injury via subtype-specific KATP channel activation and is mimicked by inhibition of the mitochondrial permeability transition pore. *Eur Heart J* 32, 1266-1274.

Park JW, Kang JW, Jeon WJ & Na HS. (2010). Postconditioning protects skeletal muscle from ischemia-reperfusion injury. *Microsurgery* 30, 223-229.

Pipinos, II, Judge AR, Selsby JT, Zhu Z, Swanson SA, Nella AA & Dodd SL. (2008a). The myopathy of peripheral arterial occlusive disease: Part 2. Oxidative stress, neuropathy, and shift in muscle fiber type. *Vasc Endovascular Surg* 42, 101-112.

Pipinos, II, Judge AR, Zhu Z, Selsby JT, Swanson SA, Johanning JM, Baxter BT, Lynch TG & Dodd SL. (2006). Mitochondrial defects and oxidative damage in patients with peripheral arterial disease. *Free Radic Biol Med* 41, 262-269.

Pipinos, II, Sharov VG, Shepard AD, Anagnostopoulos PV, Katsamouris A, Todor A, Filis KA & Sabbah HN. (2003). Abnormal mitochondrial respiration in skeletal muscle in patients with peripheral arterial disease. *J Vasc Surg* 38, 827-832.

Pipinos, II, Shepard AD, Anagnostopoulos PV, Katsamouris A & Boska MD. (2000). Phosphorus 31 nuclear magnetic resonance spectroscopy suggests a mitochondrial defect in claudicating skeletal muscle. *J Vasc Surg* 31, 944-952.

Pipinos, II, Swanson SA, Zhu Z, Nella AA, Weiss DJ, Gutti TL, McComb RD, Baxter BT, Lynch TG & Casale GP. (2008b). Chronically ischemic mouse skeletal muscle exhibits myopathy in association with mitochondrial dysfunction and oxidative damage. *Am J Physiol Regul Integr Comp Physiol* 295, R290-296.

Quinzii CM, Lopez LC, Von-Moltke J, Naini A, Krishna S, Schuelke M, Salviati L, Navas P, DiMauro S & Hirano M. (2008). Respiratory chain dysfunction and oxidative stress correlate with severity of primary CoQ10 deficiency. *FASEB J* 22, 1874-1885.

Quistorff B, Johansen L & Sahlin K. (1993). Absence of phosphocreatine resynthesis in human calf muscle during ischaemic recovery. *Biochem J* 291 (Pt 3), 681-686.

Riganti C, Gazzano E, Polimeni M, Costamagna C, Bosia A & Ghigo D. (2004). Diphenyleneiodonium inhibits the cell redox metabolism and induces oxidative stress. *J Biol Chem* 279, 47726-47731.

Rodrigues L, Crisostomo J, Matafome P, Louro T, Nunes E & Seica R. (2011). Dietary restriction improves systemic and muscular oxidative stress in type 2 diabetic Goto-Kakizaki rats. *J Physiol Biochem*.

Skyschally A, van Caster P, Iliodromitis EK, Schultz R, Kremastinos DT & Heusch G. (2009). Ischemic postconditionong: experimental models and protocol algorythms. *Basic Res Cardiol* 104, 469)483.

Sjostrom M, Angquist KA & Rais O. (1980). Intermittent claudication and muscle fiber fine structure: correlation between clinical and morphological data. *Ultrastruct Pathol* 1, 309-326.

St-Pierre J, Buckingham JA, Roebuck SJ & Brand MD. (2002). Topology of superoxide production from different sites in the mitochondrial electron transport chain. *J Biol Chem* 277, 44784-44790.

Szijarto A, Gyurkovics E, Aranyi P, Onody P, Stangl R, Tatrai M, Lotz G, Mihaly Z, Hegedus V, Blazovics A & Kupcsulijk P. (2009). Effect of postconditioning in major vascular operations on rats. *Magy Seb* 62,180-187.

Thaveau F, Zoll J, Rouyer O, Chakfé N, Kretz JG, Piquard F & Geny B. (2007). Ischemic preconditioning specifically restores complexes I and II activities of the mitochondrial respiratory chain in ischemic skeletal muscle. *J Vasc Surg* 46,541-547.

Thaveau F, Zoll J, Bouitbir J, N'Guessan B, Plobner P, Chakfe N, Kretz JG, Richard R, Piquard F & Geny B. (2010). Effect of chronic pre-treatment with angiotensin converting enzyme inhibition on skeletal muscle mitochondrial recovery after ischemia/reperfusion. *Fundam Clin Pharmacol* 24, 333-340.

Tran TP, Tu H, Pipinos, II, Muelleman RL, Albadawi H & Li YL. (2011). Tourniquet-induced acute ischemia-reperfusion injury in mouse skeletal muscles: Involvement of superoxide. *Eur J Pharmacol* 650, 328-334.

Tsubota H, Marui A, Esaki J, Bir SC, Ikeda T & Sakata R. (2010). Remote postconditioning may attenuate ischaemia-reperfusion injury in the murine hindlimb through adenosine receptor activation. *Eur J Vasc Endovasc Surg* 40, 804-809.

Turrens JF. (2003). Mitochondrial formation of reactive oxygen species. *J Physiol* 552, 335-344.

Ubbink DT & Koopman B. (2006). Near-infrared spectroscopy in the routine diagnostic work-up of patients with leg ischaemia. *Eur J Vasc Endovasc Surg* 31, 394-400.

Veksler VI, Kuznetsov AV, Sharov VG, Kapelko VI & Saks VA. (1987). Mitochondrial respiratory parameters in cardiac tissue: a novel method of assessment by using saponin-skinned fibers. *Biochim Biophys Acta* 892, 191-196.

Votyakova TV & Reynolds IJ. (2001). DeltaPsi(m)-Dependent and -independent production of reactive oxygen species by rat brain mitochondria. *J Neurochem* 79, 266-277.

Wallace DC. (2000). Mitochondrial defects in cardiomyopathy and neuromuscular disease. *Am Heart J* 139, S70-85.

Watanabe T, Matsushita M, Nishikimi N, Sakurai T, Komori K & Nimura Y. (2004). Near-infrared spectroscopy with treadmill exercise to assess lower limb ischemia in patients with atherosclerotic occlusive disease. *Surg Today* 34, 849-854.

Wredenberg A, Wibom R, Wilhelmsson H, Graff C, Wiener HH, Burden SJ, Oldfors A, Westerblad H & Larsson NG. (2002). Increased mitochondrial mass in mitochondrial myopathy mice. *Proc Natl Acad Sci U S A* 99, 15066-15071.

Zatina MA, Berkowitz HD, Gross GM, Maris JM & Chance B. (1986). 31P nuclear magnetic resonance spectroscopy: noninvasive biochemical analysis of the ischemic extremity. *J Vasc Surg* 3, 411-420.